Introduction

I practiced holistic medicine for nearly thirty-five years and this book is an attempt to recount just a few of the many very memorable experiences I had in dealing with patients. Holistic medicine treats patients by attention to the whole person: their body, mind, spirit, emotions, and even their belief system. It also involves a belief in the innate healing powers of humans. These powers have evolved over countless millennia whereas most medicines have only been around for less than 100 years.

My work was never boring. Rather, it was thrilling, exciting, and challenging because I always felt it was not a sore throat or an earache that I was seeing, but a person with that problem at that moment. And people are endlessly interesting and endlessly grateful to have you interested in them. Let me tell you how it all came to be for me.

Upon graduation from middle school, all students are required to make a selection as to which program to follow in high school. The choice is between an academic, college bound program or a commercial program to prepare to eventually enter the work force. Having graduated from a rapid advance class where we skipped two grades, all my classmates selected the academic program but I chose to matriculate in the commercial program. Both of my parents were immigrants and believed that the proper course for a female child was to graduate from high school and enter the typing pool until they settled down into marriage and raised a family. My older sister followed this route without question and I felt that since that was expected of me, I chose the program that would prepare me for that.

School started and I became involved in classes that taught bookkeeping, stenography, and typing. However, several weeks or so after the semester started, a teacher from the middle school called my parents to tell them that I belonged in an academic program and that I should switch out of the commercial program. My parents had their own struggles at that time, and as this was a small problem in relation to what they were dealing with, they really didn't care much either way. So they turned to me and asked me what I wanted to do. Since I was already missing all my friends I said I wanted to switch to the academic program and quickly applied to the school to do that.

In middle school I was voted the prettiest, and upon graduation from high school I was voted most popular. I didn't acquire those titles by being a studious nerd. Actually, I was not a serious student at all and was more interested in dating and going to parties.

Since I was only sixteen when I graduated from high school, I was too young to enter the workforce which, for most positions, required that I be at least eighteen. My parents knew that and so indulged my desire to go on to college since there was virtually no reasonable alternative. It definitely helped that college was free and just a short bus ride away with a five cent fare.

The first two years of college consisted of all liberal arts courses, but by the third year we were asked to declare our major course of study. Compelled to make a decision, I chose to be pre-med because that's where all the boys were. I was by then only about eighteen and still not a very serious student. However, in the fourth and last year of college, reality bit and I realized that the parents who barely indulged my desire to go to college at all, were certainly not going to see me through medical school. So, I quickly signed up for courses in the education department which would prepare me to become a teacher. Upon graduation I was offered a job in a middle school in the lower east side of Manhattan. That area was considered to be a ghetto and the schools had a very difficult time acquiring and keeping teachers. Since one year of education courses was not sufficient to qualify me for a teaching license I was granted a provisional license because the school was so desperate for a teacher, particularly one with a science background.

I started teaching at that school and quickly realized that I was committed to a place that made the book "The Blackboard Jungle" seem like a nursery rhyme. Leaving, however, was not an option since the provisional teaching license didn't qualify me to teach elsewhere. After about a year and a half at that school, I suddenly came down with a serious illness called Crohn's disease. Crohn's disease has a wide spectrum of severity and I was at the worst end. I was admitted to the hospital with a fever of 106 and was immediately wrapped in ice and placed on the critical list. That hospitalization lasted seven months during which I had to have life-saving surgery. Upon discharge from the hospital I was sent to a rehabilitation facility and spent another three months there. Finally I went back home but had a number of relapses which put me back in the hospital again. During the next eight years I had numerous hospitalizations and surgeries. Finally I began to recover and was able to return to work and other life activities. I married and had two children. The illness was a life-changing event, and I was no longer the fun-loving, empty-headed party girl. I had a totally different perspective on life and a markedly changed value system. I also now had a wonderful husband and two rambunctious but equally wonderful sons.

While raising my children, I completed my master's degree and taught two afternoons a week at the university. One day I approached my husband and asked him if he could commit to coming home from work early on those two days that I was at the university because I wanted to take an evening class in biochemistry. He stared long and hard at me and then said that he would give me his answer in three days. I couldn't understand why he needed three days to deliver a simple yes or no and so pressured him for an immediate answer. He said no; he would give me his answer in three days. So, after three days he said yes he would come home early so that I could remain at school for the evening class. Many years later, I asked him why he needed three days to give me an answer, and he responded that he could see where all this was leading even when I couldn't. The other thing I did during this period when my children were young was to take a year of calculus on the Sunrise Semester. That was a program very early in the morning that enabled people to earn college credits after taking the course and passing the examinations which were given by a local university.

It wasn't until my own children started school that I myself could see where all this was heading. I became aware that I really had a very strong desire to become a physician and that all along, without even realizing it, the classes in biochemistry and calculus were to satisfy the prerequisites that I was missing to apply to medical school. However, I was now thirty-two years old, a wife and mother and my husband had a wonderful job in charge of the construction of what was then and still is today the largest sewage treatment plant in the world. We also owned our home which added to my lack of choice and mobility. Most applicants to medical school have the luxury of being able to pick up their toothbrush and go to wherever the school is located that accepts them. I did not have that luxury. But I knew I could never live with myself if I didn't try, so I applied to one school, once. Much to my surprise, I was granted an interview.

However, the evening before the interview, my younger son was playing out in our backyard with an older boy and got hit in the back of his head with the wooden seat of a swing. Within minutes he lost consciousness and began to have projectile vomiting. Fortunately at that time my husband came home from work, and we rushed him to the nearest hospital where a skull fracture was diagnosed. Since he was comatose and unresponsive, he was admitted to the hospital. This was in the day before accommodations for parents were made in the pediatric wards of hospitals, and my husband and I slept the night on the concrete floor of our son's hospital room, alternating getting up to check on him.

The next morning I called to cancel my interview at the medical school, telling them what happened to my son. In my wildest dreams I never thought I would ever be granted another interview. The nurses came in to check on my son's mental status every few hours, but he remained unresponsive for four more days. Finally, after four days, he opened his eyes but still did not speak. The nurses kept coming into the room saying to him "wake up little boy, what is your name, what is your name?" I guess he didn't like being constantly awakened and annoyed by them, and so he finally responded in an angry tone, "My name is nobody". Everyone breathed a heaping sigh of relief and we knew we had our little boy back. His roommate was an eight-year-old boy who would, without any provocation, suddenly utter vulgar expletives. As he did that, he would put his hands on his neck as if trying to stop the words. But they came out anyway, and he seemed not to be able to keep himself from doing that. His behavior created in me an immense desire to understand what caused him to do that and how he could be helped. I also noted that the staff never tried to punish or control him when he did that, and that they treated him as a sick boy, rather than a bad one. However, as my main focus at the time was on my son's recovery, I soon forgot about the other boy. My son spent a few more days in the hospital, and then we took him home. He made a rapid recovery and even now has never sustained any lasting effects from the event.

And surprise of surprises, I was granted another interview at the medical school.

Not having very high hopes of acceptance as I realized I had too many strikes against me, I nevertheless went for the interview. The interviewer was smoking a pipe as I entered as this was in the days before smoking in offices was prohibited. He barely glanced in my direction as he looked at my records and letters of recommendation. Finally he looked up and asked me this question: "Tell me why, as we receive thousands of applications from equally qualified people, why should we accept you with your 'encumbrances'?" I knew he was referring to my children as "encumbrances" so I responded, "It is precisely because of those 'encumbrances' that I will be a wonderful physician."

He didn't seem too impressed with my answer, and the interview soon ended as there was a long line in the waiting room yet to be interviewed.

However, several weeks later, my acceptance letter came in the mail. It was originally my intention to become a pathologist as I enjoyed looking at slides of tissues and making the diagnosis from what I saw. I had had several courses in this in college and found it very interesting and did very well in the exams. The first two years of medical school are all academic, but in the third year we begin to do our clinical clerkships in the hospitals and for the first time come in contact with patients. I found that I also very much enjoyed interacting with people and started to have second thoughts about being a pathologist. The more contact I had with patients the more I thought about becoming a primary care physician. I found I had good communication skills, and since I felt I knew medicine from both sides of the bed from my own experience with a serious illness, I could empathize with the patients and had a more intimate knowledge of their needs and how best to serve them.

I recalled that during my own hospitalization, frequently when the doctors came into my room while on their rounds, they would stand often at the entrance to the door and say something like "so how are we doing today?" Since I always felt that their body language conveyed to me that they didn't have time for any elaborate responses, I always responded, "Just fine." But how "fine" could I have been after all those months in the hospital on the critical list? After that, I always made it my policy when visiting a patient in the hospital to sit down with them on the chair next to their bedside. That body language, I felt, sent the message that I was interested in and had the time to listen to what they had to tell me. It was also during these first patient experiences that I encountered another patient who also suffered from uncontrollable vulgar utterances. I learned that he had Tourette's syndrome and recalled that was what the little boy who shared the hospital room with my son years before suffered from.

One day one of the professors was talking informally to the class and made a remark which stuck in my mind even to today. He told us that it cost society $53,000 a year to educate each and every one of us. My tuition was only $1,000 a year. That left in me a very strong feeling that I owed a debt to society which I had an obligation to return. I developed the feeling that I could most effectively return this debt to society by becoming a Family Physician which at that moment I decided to do. Although I knew at the time that Family Practice was probably the least lucrative of all the medical specialties, I nevertheless chose to do it as I knew it was where I could be the most effective and gain the most satisfaction.

Upon graduation I entered a Family Practice residency, and that is what I did when I opened my office upon completion. I never looked back. I loved being involved with people and always felt privileged that they felt confident enough in me to trust my judgment in determining what was best for their health and safety. In quite a few cases, I took care of all the members of a family. At first I would only see the mothers and the children as the fathers were not comfortable with a female physician, but that changed in time. With some patients I was in the delivery room at their birth and many years later did their premarital physicals. For some reason, I had the uncanny ability to remember details of their lives when even they didn't remember them themselves. I once asked a friend why I was able to do this. She replied, "Because you care about them so much." Yes, I did care very much about them.

In the early years of my medical practice, there were times that I had to refer a patient to a specialist. Often, then, I would withdraw from their case, assuming the specialist knew a lot more than I about the problem and I no longer had anything to offer.

One day I was reading a medical magazine and was struck by an article about recovery from a heart attack. The article reported an extensive study which concluded that the two most important factors in recovery in the first twenty-four hours after a heart attack were:

1. Whether they were attended to in a hospital equipped and experienced in dealing with the problem and
2. Whether they had been visited by their Family Physician.

This had a tremendous impact on me and my subsequent involvement in cases where I had to refer the patient to a specialist. From then on, I remained intimately involved in the case with both the specialist and the patient and never again belittled the role I had to play. I found this newly adopted attitude paid off in a multitude of ways. Countless times patients would call me after a visit with the specialist and ask, "So what did he say?" And, because I now was intimately involved, I was able to answer their question in terms that they could understand, which, at times, either the specialist was unable to do or the patient's anxiety kept them from understanding.

The hospital where I was on staff had an alcohol and drug rehabilitation unit, but it was not housed at the acute care campus but on another campus which was several miles away. Many patients that were admitted to the unit had accompanying medical problems requiring immediate care. The nurses would call the acute care hospital to request the services of one of the physicians to assist with the management of the patient. Most of the doctors didn't really care to respond as it took quite a bit of time out of a busy day to leave the main campus, get in their car and drive to the other campus just to see one patient. And since many of the patients were indigents and didn't have medical insurance, the doctors often did not get paid. However, I went every time I was called and in turn received the reward for good work which was more work.

It didn't take too long before I was the one getting called much of the time and found myself spending quite a bit of time on the unit and getting to know the patients and their families as well. I was often very impressed with my observation that the alcoholics and addicts, when sober, were quite extraordinary people. I recalled reading once that a very significant number of Nobel Prize winners were addicted people, so this was not that much of a surprise to me. However, I also could not help noticing that there was a constellation of people surrounding them that had suffered a great deal because of their connection to the addict. I found myself getting very interested in the field and started to attend some open twelve-step meetings. After a while I decided to get more training in the new field of Addiction Medicine and took classes to acquire certification. That also required doing a fellowship at an alcohol and drug hospital, and I arranged for someone to cover my practice while I took a leave of absence to do it. I felt I also needed more background in psychology and so I signed up for a second master's degree to attain that. I also attended evening classes at a Psychoanalytic Institute to further my education in that field. It took two years of hard work, but I became certified as a specialist in Addiction Medicine and was the first person to be listed in the Yellow Pages in that field.

When I returned to my office, I continued my work as a Family Practice Physician, but also saw patients with addiction problems—and their families—in my office. In time, as I became known in the area, my practice expanded to people with other addictions who also came in for treatment. My practice began to expand to people with addiction to eating, gambling, sex, and even spending. Significant others required treatment as well, as they were often as sick as the addicts. In fact, in many cases they were harder to treat, as many of them subscribed to the belief that "what's wrong with me is you". It was often difficult to get them to believe that they too were sick and needed treatment. That is why twelve-step groups called Al-Anon were started to help them.

I loved being involved with the addicts and their significant others, although I must admit the success rate was not that high, and even when successful, there was a considerable relapse rate. However, when successful, it was very gratifying not only to see the addict's life turned around but also the lives of the constellation of people that were affected by them.

The Family Physician has a unique role to play which is different from the experience of the specialist. I often took care of all the members of a family, and so when one came in with a problem I always felt that I needed to be cognizant of what was going on with the entire family. I did a lot of infant care, and since much of it—such as height, weight, and immunizations—can be attended to by a staff member, I tried to concentrate more on and be aware of parent-child interactions because much later psychopathology has its origins in infancy. So, I asked questions regarding family support, and issues involving toilet training and sibling interactions. Toilet training itself is a fascinating issue since it is the first activity that the child, not the parent, can control. Many parents intervene to reestablish the control and resort to methods that can have long-lasting deleterious effects on the child.

One day a mother brought an infant for a well baby check up at 11 A.M. I couldn't help noticing that the mother smelled strongly of alcohol and quickly realized that the patient that required more of my attention this day was the mother and not the infant. So here was another instance where my role as the Family Physician led me to direct my attention not only to the patient in front of me, but also to the family member who brought them in.

I did not choose retirement; retirement chose me. I developed a spinal problem which had me hospitalized and then housebound for nine months. After that time all the patients had been reassigned to other doctors, and I would have gone back to an empty office to start over. The Bible says "for all things there is a season", and I concluded it was my season to retire. People ask me if I miss my medical practice. I must admit it is nice not to have to get up at 3 A.M. and go to the ER, but I do miss my patients and the families I was involved with for so many years. I always felt privileged that they chose me to serve them, and I always did that to the best of my ability.

In retirement I moved to Florida and took up new hobbies of learning the piano, painting, and playing bridge, all of which I enjoy very much. In 2017 someone anonymously submitted my name to enter the Ms. Senior Florida Pageant. I didn't know anything about the pageant, but I read the mandate, which was to celebrate senior women who, after not being any longer involved with work or child-rearing, had reinvented their lives in creative and productive ways. This very much impressed me. So I agreed to participate and much to my surprise won the pageant to represent the state as Ms. Senior Florida. As a senior woman I was proud to be selected to serve as an example of what the pageant represented. Afterward they sent me to Atlantic City, New Jersey, to represent the state of Florida in the Ms. Senior American Pageant. That was a totally extraordinary experience as I got to meet so many senior women from all over the country who were all actively devoting their lives to creative and productive activities.

I decided to write this book to share the immense satisfaction I had in helping others and to provide an example of the many rewards of choosing Family Practice as a specialty. I hope that you will find it interesting and informative and that my story will attract others to embark on this glorious and noble journey.

Contents

❦

Andy

⌒⌒⌒

Early one morning I was reading the newspaper with my breakfast, and my attention was immediately captured by an article on the front page. It was about a truck driver who had accidentally killed a thirteen-year-old boy on a bicycle. According to the story, the boy had suddenly come out into the street from between two cars which was why he was not seen by the truck driver until it was too late. As I read further, I saw that the driver was a patient of mine and I did the care for him and his wife and child. I recalled that his child was also a thirteen-year-old boy, and so I knew that this would have an especially strong impact on my patient Andy, the driver of the truck. I knew the family well and knew that Andy was a responsible person and that he did not have any problem with alcohol or drugs.

I recalled that the year before, Andy's son, Robert, had been bitten by a rattlesnake and nearly died. They lived out in a secluded, densely wooded area because Andy had a taxidermy hobby and that area provided easily obtainable specimens for him. The son had been hunting in the woods with his father and unearthed a clump of brush when a rattlesnake suddenly sprung out and bit him on the arm. He cried out and Andy came to him, saw the bite marks on his arm and immediately fashioned a tourniquet above the wound. Within minutes Robert began to have difficulty breathing and fainted. Andy scooped him up in his arms and started to run out of the woods seeking help. It took about another fifteen minutes to get to a phone and call 911 and another ten minutes or so before an ambulance arrived. Thirty minutes is considered a critical time to get help, and they were already past that point. By the time Robert got to the hospital, he had stopped breathing and had to be given artificial respiration.

In the hospital, rattlesnake antivenom was immediately administered, and Robert was intubated and put on a ventilator and transferred to the Intensive Care Unit. It was fortunate that the hospital had a supply of antivenom on hand—as being surrounded by wooded areas which attracted numerous hikers, snake bites were not all that uncommon.

The hospital called to tell me what had happened, and I immediately rushed to the ICU. I met with Andy, and, as his wife Sarah had been called at her work, she immediately rushed to the hospital. They were extremely distraught and although I tried to assure them that he would receive the best of care where he was, they could not hold back their tears and they both sobbed uncontrollably.

Robert had a stormy course in the Intensive Care Unit and required medications to support his blood pressure. However, after several days on the ventilator, Robert's vital signs began to improve, and he was able to come off respiratory support. His condition continued to improve, and after a week he was able to be discharged to his home. He was left with a numb lower arm around the snake bite which was caused by the snake venom which was toxic to the nerves. In time, that numbness lessened as his nerves began to recover. He is still left with some numbness but fortunately has full use of his arm and fingers.

I felt a great sadness as I read the newspaper article knowing what distress it brought, both to the parents of the boy that was struck and killed, and also to Andy. Although he was not prosecuted and blamed, I knew Andy would suffer greatly too with the recollection of the tragedy.

I did not think again of the incident until about nine months later when Andy's wife Sarah came to the office with a minor ailment. Her presence jogged my memory, and I asked her how Andy was doing. That question unleashed a torrent of tears through which she told me that Andy was doing terribly. She told me that he said he could never return to being a truck driver again and that he was home now all the time. Her meager salary was the only support the family had, and her job did not include health insurance for the family. She also told me that he is up and just paces the floor night after night. I told her to tell Andy to come in to see me as I felt he might need someone to talk to, but she said that without insurance coverage they could not afford any additional fees. I told her not to worry about that and that I would see him and try to help him at no charge. She said she would tell him that, but, knowing them, I suspected they were too proud to accept the help.

So he did not come in at that time, but did come in about six months later. I was happy to see him looking well and smiling. When I asked him what was going on he told me that when he could no longer return to being a truck driver he started doing his taxidermy hobby in earnest and apparently had gained a reputation in the area and had recently won some awards. That led to being contacted by someone who was planning a safari to Africa and wanted to be accompanied by a taxidermist. Apparently, as Andy told me, animals are better preserved if they can be treated right after the kill rather than being frozen and brought back to the states to be mounted. So, because of his recently acquired reputation in the field, he told me the man had contacted him and offered to take him on the safari all expenses paid. Andy grinned from ear to ear as he related this story and explained that he was getting to realize the dream of his lifetime.

Before going on a safari or any trip to a malaria-ridden area, one should take prophylactic antimalarial medication and continue it after the trip is completed. So, I gave Andy a prescription for the medication and cheerfully sent him on his way.

Three weeks later, Andy showed up again in my office. I immediately noticed that this time he didn't look too happy as he was covered head to toe with a really angry looking rash. He said it had started while he was over in Africa and since medical care was not readily available he decided to come back home. Fortunately the safari had been completed and the man was pleased and satisfied with his catch and the treatment that Andy had administered. The man even said he would like to hire Andy again to accompany him on more hunts for wild animals.

I looked over Andy's rash carefully and then asked him whether he wanted the good news or the bad news first. He chose the bad news, and I told him I was not certain what was causing this terribly severe rash. The same rash can have a multitude of causations, and I didn't know which it was. The good news, however, was that I could probably treat it anyway. I told him we would give my treatment about two days to see if it was effective, and if not, that I would have to send him to New York University's Center for Tropical Medicine where they deal with obscure and unusual tropical diseases which Andy may have sustained out in the wild.

So, I prescribed what I thought would work and made an appointment for him to return in two days. He came in and I could see that the rash seemed to be about 50 percent better. I told him to continue with the medication that I had prescribed and see me again in several days. Again he returned, and now I could see he was nearly all better.

With a lot of dermatologic diseases, the causes never turned up, but they often can be treated anyway. I never did know what caused that severe rash in Andy's case, but I was pleased to see him get better and not have it recur. I did consider the possibility that this could have been an allergic reaction to the antimalarial medication so when he needed it once again for future safaris, I prescribed something different.

I continued to see Andy and his family for a number of years until my own retirement. Although Andy never forgot the terrible tragedy which had so altered his own life, it was pleasing to me to see the delight he was getting from his new career as a renowned taxidermist. He had gained a considerable following in the field and was getting many requests for his services.

After he left, I thought to myself that sometimes out of the worst things that can happen in life, can come the best.

MaryAnn

ल◌ৎ৩ঔ

My husband had recently heard from a friend that had successfully quit smoking. His friend had been a two pack a day smoker for many years, but after hearing from his doctor that he had developed COPD (chronic obstructive pulmonary disease), he realized he needed to quit smoking or would soon be crippled by the disease. Actually, as he later related to my husband, he didn't need the doctor to tell him that. For some time he had been noticing that he had difficulty catching his breath with even small exertions.

My own husband was also a two pack a day smoker. I was a smoker as well, but had quit seventeen years before—in medical school. While taking class in gross anatomy where we dissected cadavers, I saw the effects of smoking on the lungs. My team's cadaver had black lungs and had been a smoker, but the cadaver on the neighboring table had pink lungs and probably had not been a smoker. Seeing that makes a stark impression on the students, and at that time they all quit. Although some eventually gravitated back to smoking, I never did.

My husband had made numerous attempts to quit smoking but had not been successful. In withdrawal, he would get very anxious and pace the floor continuously. Each time he was so distressed he gave up the attempt.

However, when he learned of his friend's success in quitting, and knowing that with prior attempts his friend had similarly suffered and been unsuccessful, he decided to find out how his friend managed to be successful this time. He learned that his friend had had ear acupuncture and that the treatment made for a much more comfortable and easy withdrawal.

So my husband sought out the same doctor that treated his friend and had a staple put in his ear. I couldn't believe what I was seeing in the days after the treatment. My husband was calm and comfortable and seemed to have no desire to have a cigarette. If there was any side effect at all, it was that my husband was taking short naps through the day, something which he had never done before. The treatment consisted of having the staple in for one month but because I was so delighted with the success, I urged him to keep it in and not rush to remove it. He kept it in for nine months and never smoked again.

I was so impressed with his and his friend's success I decided it was something I should look into as it might be a useful addition to my work with addicts. So I made inquiries and learned of a physician at a hospital in New York City that was having a lot of success with the technique. I contacted him, and he invited me to come to a clinic he held at the hospital and if I wished, he would be happy to train me and tell me how to order supplies.

I attended his clinic the following week, which was held at a hospital in Harlem in New York City. The hospital was in the midst of a ghetto area and attracted mostly indigent patients. When I arrived at the information desk to learn where the clinic was, I was directed to a large meeting room about the size of a gymnasium. Upon entering, I immediately noticed that it was filled with hundreds of people all seated around the perimeter of the room. The quiet in the room surprised me, especially as I learned that most of the people in the room were criminals and had been remanded there by the courts to receive treatment for their drug addiction and dealing, as an alternative to incarceration. I also noticed that everyone seemed calm and many were conversing quietly. There was also a lot of friendly hugging that was going on. Dr. Smith noticed my arrival and came to greet me. I watched him giving ear acupuncture treatments to a number of people, which required insertion of very fine needles into several areas in the outer part of their ear. The patients were all very thankful and said they were grateful for the treatment and that it was effective in curbing their desire for street drugs. Many of the patients had family members with them, who also seemed very happy with the success of the treatment.

I met with Dr. Smith several more times and then when I felt confident about doing it, I started to perform the treatment with some of my addict patients. At first I only did it with smokers. I also learned that an apparatus had recently been invented that could detect the location of the acupuncture points more precisely making unnecessary the insertion of numerous needles to increase the success of finding the proper point. This made it easier on the patient and was also more cosmetically acceptable. I ordered tiny needles which were held in place by a flesh colored sticky tape and were barely noticeable. Patients then could go about their normal lives for weeks with the pin in place and without attracting attention.

As word got out, numerous patients flocked to my office for the treatment. I couldn't believe how successful it was. Although acupuncture has been used in the Far East for thousands of years, no one really knew why or how it works. I can only say that, for many of my patients, it worked.

One day a lady named MaryAnn came into my office. She related that she had been referred to me by her pulmonologist because he was very concerned about her deteriorating lung function. At that time she was smoking two packs of cigarettes a day. She told me that she had tried many times before to quit smoking but found withdrawal so uncomfortable she could never be successful for long. She also said that she heard that two of her friends had been successful with my ear acupuncture treatments and that she wanted to give that a try.

I inserted the staple and directed her to return in three days when I would remove the staple and place another in her other ear. I learned that after a few days the stimulation waned and so I would change the point to gain renewed stimulation again. As time went on, with ongoing success, the treatments lessened, but in some cases went on for months.

I was delighted with MaryAnn's success and so was she. She reported feeling much better; she was coughing a lot less, and I noted that she also looked a lot better. She had good color and looked a lot less haggard. Although she was in her forties, she could easily have been mistaken for someone in their sixties as her smoking habit created a lot of wrinkles in her skin and aged her prematurely. I kept seeing her weekly for several months until we both felt she didn't require the treatments any longer.

About six months later, I saw MaryAnn again in my office for her yearly physical. She had at that point been completely off cigarettes for about ten months. At the visit she informed me that she had made arrangements to realize the dream of her lifetime which was to make a trip to Machu

Picchu in the mountains of Peru. She was to leave the following week. I grew quite concerned at this news because I knew of the elevation of the site and didn't think her lung function could tolerate the thinned air. Even healthy people are advised to undergo a period of acclimatization before ascending to such heights, and to make a gradual ascent over several weeks. I also knew that to get there, the flight landed at an airport at an even higher elevation. In time, most patients experience improved lung function after they quit smoking and even have a reduced risk for lung cancer. However, that only happens—if it happens at all—after many years of smoking sobriety. I felt it was much too soon for MaryAnn to take that risk. I told her what I felt, and she was shocked and dismayed to hear this. She even seemed to become somewhat annoyed with me and said that she saw her pulmonologist the week before and when she told him of her intended trip, he didn't say anything. I said that might be because he did not realize the elevation of the tourist site. I acquainted her with the dangers, but could see that my warnings were not making any inroads.

About a month later she came back into my office again, to be checked for what she told me was a recent case of pneumonia from which she was recovering. She then related to me the story of what happened to her on her trip to Machu Picchu.

As the plane flew into the airport at Cusco, which is at an elevation of nearly 11,000 feet, she began to feel short of breath and fainted. The flight attendants arranged for an ambulance to be waiting at the airport. Upon arrival she was taken to a hospital and had to be put on very high flow oxygen. It was decided by the doctors that that was no place for a person with such severe lung dysfunction and so she was taken by helicopter to a hospital at lower altitude. While there she developed a pneumonia, likely because her severely weakened state did not permit her to cough effectively. She remained at that hospital in their Intensive Care Unit for two weeks and was finally able to fly home. Even for the flight home she required a portable oxygen supply.

MaryAnn finally recovered and was able to return to her work as a flower arranger at a local florist. I go into the shop occasionally when I need flowers for a special occasion. I am always delighted to see MaryAnn looking so much better and hearing her news that she is still able to remain off cigarettes. In fact, she says she is now repulsed when she sees someone smoking and cannot stand the smell of their smoke.

It is gratifying to see now so many restrictions about smoking in public places. But this was a long time coming. Even after the Surgeon General of the United States, Dr. Everett Kopp, warned in 1964 about the dangers of smoking, it took at least another generation before the danger of exposure to secondhand smoke was realized.

The hospital where I was on staff permitted smoking all over the hospital for about another thirty years. For many years I constantly made a fuss about the prevalence of smoke at meetings and in patient's rooms, offices, and the hospital cafeteria. I frequently would point out at meetings how hypocritical it was to be treating people for the ravages of smoking while permitting it to occur all over the hospital. Often, I would noisily stomp out of a meeting but not before making a strong statement about my unwillingness to breathe all the smoke that so many were generating by smoking in my presence.

However, in the 1990's, evidence began to emerge about the danger of secondhand smoke and little by little hospitals around the country were starting to go smoke free. So our hospital decided to form a committee to get our hospital smoke free. And guess who they put in charge of the committee. Me, the gadfly.

The committee decided it would be done gradually. So, little by little, areas of the hospital became smoke free. The entire process took two years. It was decided that the last areas would be the psychiatric unit and the alcohol and drug rehabilitation unit as a lot of resistance was anticipated. The hospital even feared it would lose patients by instituting the policy. Since at the time I was spending a lot of time at the alcohol and drug unit, I was well positioned to observe how it all went. Much to everyone's surprise, it went very smoothly.

I guess decisions in life are much easier to make when there is no choice.

Today, there are many fewer smokers in our country than there were. I credit this to increased restrictions on smoking in public places and more available information on the dangers of smoking as well as exposure to secondhand smoke. The increased tax, which has greatly elevated the cost of a pack of cigarettes, has no doubt played a role as well.

However, there is now increased use of electronic cigarettes, which are being aggressively marketed to our youth. It has also been recently discovered that, although these cigarettes were touted as being much safer, they are not really so and carry their own dangers.

New laws are being placed on the books to regulate them more carefully. However, the lobbying market is quite powerful, and I suspect they will be around for quite a while yet. I suppose so long as there is money to be made on something there will always be people around to snare the vulnerable. And vulnerable they are. Cigarette smoking has been likened by many to be as compelling an addiction as heroin.

Frank

❦

On a Friday evening as I was preparing to go to bed in the hope of getting some sleep, I was shaken out of that fantasy by the jarring ring of the telephone. As I was covering three busy practices that weekend, I knew before picking up the phone that it definitely wasn't a social call.

It was a call from the Emergency Room of the hospital where I had been on staff for the past fifteen years. The nurse in charge described a patient that had been brought to the ER a short while ago by his family. The brief history the nurse gave me was of a thirty-two-year-old strapping man who was brought in by his family because of the sudden onset of wild, belligerent, totally out of control behavior. According to the family, he and his four children had been shopping at a local mall just earlier that evening and there were no signs at all of this behavior nor had he ever exhibited behavior like this before. The first thought of the ER staff was of drug usage but his wife swore up and down that he was not a drug user and had never been one. She said he wouldn't even take an aspirin if he had a headache. The staff had been unable to even take his vital signs because he was thrashing about so violently.

I got dressed again and headed to the ER shortly thereafter. It was a very foggy evening, and I drove slowly, not certain if it was the fog or a sense of foreboding about the patient I was going to attend to. If the staff couldn't deal with him, I wondered how I could.

I parked and as I approached the entrance to the ER, I was aware of loud shouts inside. Upon entering, I immediately noted a large gathering around one of the rooms, with several family members standing outside looking extremely distressed and anxious. The head nurse saw me, rolled her eyes, and pointed to the door of the room where the crowd was gathered. Upon entering I recognized several of the hospital security guards who were engaged—not very successfully—in holding the patient down. No one had been able to take the patient's vital signs but someone did manage to slip a thermometer under the patient's armpit without him noticing, where it was noted he had a temperature of 104 degrees Fahrenheit. This finding quickly shifted my thinking away from drug usage to a possible case of meningitis. I knew a spinal tap would have to be done to confirm my suspicion but how to accomplish this on a patient who was thrashing about so violently?

As I pondered this question, I noticed that one of the neurologists was seeing another patient in the ER and so I approached him and asked him to help me. We agreed that the only way a spinal tap could be safely done was to administer a short acting paralytic drug which we requested the nursing staff acquire from the hospital pharmacy. This was not an easy task as the hospital pharmacy had only a skeleton staff at that hour and asked us to substantiate our need for such an infrequently used drug. That finally accomplished, I approached the patient's wife to tell her of our plan and to obtain some more history on the patient. About all I could get from her was that he was very healthy, had never been ill, and was currently a local hero for numerous sports-related accomplishments.

We administered the drug by injection and were grateful the needle didn't break inside him. The drug began to take effect in the next few minutes, and he became still, although alert and aware of what was happening to him. With the help of several nurses brought in to assist us, we gloved up and the spinal tap was accomplished without event.

Spinal fluid is usually clear, but it was immediately apparent that his fluid looked like milk which added to my strong suspicion of a case of meningitis. The milky look, I suspected, was caused by large numbers of white cells in his spinal fluid, signaling a severe infection. We sent the specimen off to the lab requesting a stat result. The patient was transferred to a room in the isolation area of the hospital and tied to the bed with strong straps as the paralytic was already wearing off.

The first result on the spinal fluid arrived within thirty minutes and the reading was that it contained 42,000 white cells per millimeter. A note was appended to the lab result that said that that was the highest white count that had ever been reported in spinal fluid in that hospital.

I knew this was a very ominous sign. I really didn't expect this patient to survive, and I thought that if he did, he would probably have very significant neurologic impairment. The specimen was also sent for cultures to determine what was the virulent germ that had caused this extremely severe infection in such a short time, and what antibiotics it would be sensitive to. But those results would not be available for another forty-eight hours, so we had to treat the patient empirically until they were available. The neurologist and I agreed that to provide broad coverage we would need to use very high doses of at least two broad spectrum antibiotics.

I went out to speak with the patient's wife and tell her the news while trying to be at the same time realistic about the severity of his illness but also holding out hope. I also informed her that all contacts needed to be treated immediately with a broad spectrum antibiotic to hopefully prevent them from coming down with a similar illness.

I later learned that the news about Frank's illness traveled quickly in the small town that he lived in. Also, because he was such a local hero, crowds of people just stood and sat around in the hospital lobby for the next few days waiting for news. People were so fearful that anyone who had even been in the same vicinity of Frank for the week before he fell ill, went to their doctors, insisting they received prophylactic drugs as well.

For the next few days, I visited Frank's bedside four to five times a day, not because I thought I needed to do anything for him, but to be a reassuring presence to his wife and children so they could feel he was being constantly watched and not a stone left unturned for his care.

By about the third day of antibiotic treatment when I came to Frank's bedside, I noted he was a lot more alert and calm and smiled and said "hi Doc" when I walked in. I asked him if he would like to be untied from the bed and he said yes he would, and he promised not to interfere with all the tubes going into him. His wife was smiling and so too were his four children sitting outside the room. For the first time, I felt a glimmer of optimism about his recovery.

Frank spent another fourteen days in the hospital, and each time I came I could see his improvement. By day seven he was able to get out of bed and use the bathroom. He and his wife never stopped thanking me for "saving his life," but I demurred saying it was a miracle and I couldn't take responsibility for it. They would hear none of this and kept praising me.

Frank went on to full recovery with absolutely no apparent neurologic deficits. No one else in his family took ill, and there were no reports of any similar incidents in the community. He was welcomed home by about half the town turning out with banners, music, and outdoor barbecues. I was invited but frankly felt uncomfortable with all the credit I was being given for his recovery. I mostly felt that I was little more than a bystander to nothing less than a miracle.

This story doesn't quite end here, though. Frank and his family switched to my practice, and I had contact with them for many years after. They never stopped thanking me for "saving his life" and no amount of demurring on my part made any difference.

My mother used to visit at my home and when my husband and I were out at work, she would sit on our porch. Eager for some company, she would chat with any passersby. Frank was a postman in our town but usually delivered to another part of the town. However, when our postman was off or away, Frank would deliver to our house. One day my mother was sitting outside on the porch as usual, and Frank came to deliver the mail. My mother greeted him and tells him she doesn't live here but she is my mother. He says he knows that and then tells her that her daughter saved his life. This perks up my mother considerably and she asks him to tell her what happened which he eagerly does. For years afterward, when my mother visited she would wait to see if he would deliver the mail that day which, because he was not our regular mailman, only happened once in a while. Nevertheless, rain or shine she was out there waiting for him. And, when he did come, her first question would be "so tell me what happened that night?" She never tired of hearing the story.

Edith and Cybil

❧☙

Whenever a new patient or family called the office to request that we be the providers of their medical care we always invited them to come in at no charge and meet with me at first before signing up. They were requested to bring with them any questions they might have about how to go about this, what we required, how to go about forwarding records, and, not least of all, any questions they might have about my practice habits. I would meet with them after office hours, and often we would sit together in the waiting room which was not only more spacious than the examination rooms but also more collegial and less clinical, and so made for a more friendly way of getting acquainted. I always offered this service because, if, after meeting me they had decided to go elsewhere, all the trouble involved in transferring records and arranging for ongoing care would be avoided. Fortunately, this never happened, and the patients after our meetings never decided to go elsewhere.

One cold winter afternoon, I met with the Barone family which consisted of the husband, the wife, and two teenage daughters. They told me they had recently moved into the area as the husband had been transferred in his work but also that they were particularly delighted with the move as it brought them closer to their large extended family. I asked them if there was anything particularly urgent they might like me to arrange for them and also if they had any questions for me about the conduct of my medical practice. They then told me that the older daughter, at the age of fourteen, had made a serious suicide attempt the year before and had been under the care of a psychiatrist at their former location. They asked me to refer someone in this area to continue her ongoing care. I later learned that the suicide attempt had been serious enough to put her into a coma, and that she required an exchange transfusion to save her. During an exchange transfusion the patient is hooked up to a machine which in effect washes the patient's blood of the offending agent. It is a kind of dialysis. I looked over at the older girl, Edith, and saw a lovely attractive teen who looked totally normal and happy. However, in view of the serious history, I made the referral to a trusted colleague. As both parents and the younger daughter had no significant medical history to relate, we ended our meeting cordially and they said they would make appointments soon to see me professionally.

The arrangements for the transfer of records went without event, and I saw all the family members for minor ailments now and then over the next year. Our relationship went along smoothly, and the older daughter was happy in the care of the psychiatrist I recommended and said she liked him.

However, one evening I got a call from the Emergency Room of the hospital to tell me that my patient, the younger daughter Cybil of the Barone family had made a suicide attempt earlier that evening and was brought in by ambulance, unresponsive with alarming vital signs. I was eating dinner as the call came in but immediately left the table and rushed to the hospital. I found the distraught parents in the waiting room outside the ER and was told that when they called her to come to dinner and got no response they entered her room to find her passed out with an empty bottle of Tylenol at her bedside. Since she had been in her room all afternoon where it was assumed she was doing her homework, they didn't know how long before they found her that she had ingested the pills. They also did not know how many pills were originally in the bottle.

When I entered the cubicle where she was lying, the emergency room physician was already performing a gastric lavage. This is a procedure to wash out the stomach of any pill residue to prevent further absorption. The lavage produced a small number of broken up pill material but it was suspected that more had already passed through the stomach and been absorbed since the actual time of ingestion was not known. Blood tests for acetaminophen level had already been drawn and sent, and we anxiously awaited the results. Before removing the gastric tube, a dose of activated charcoal was administered through it in the hope of preventing further absorption. Activated charcoal works by trapping toxins and chemicals in the gut by attracting the molecules to its surface and preventing their absorption. When the results of the blood tests arrived, a call was put through to the Poison Control Center to assist with the management of the case. This is routinely done in most hospitals in cases of either accidental or deliberate ingestion of harmful or harmful doses of most anything. The center is available twenty-four hours a day and is an invaluable resource as they maintain a huge list of substances and the recommended course of treatments for the management of overdoses and accidental ingestions. As always, they were a huge help to us in managing Cybil's case.

The blood results showed a markedly elevated acetaminophen level, but her liver and kidney functions were normal showing that they were not yet affected by the overdose. I went out to the parents to inform them about what was happening. However, as we kept drawing acetaminophen levels every hour and saw that they were continuing to rise, the Poison Control Center recommended we administer an antidote immediately, which we did. They also recommended she be transferred to another hospital nearby which had a pediatric intensive care unit and the capability to perform an exchange transfusion, if required. So, I placed the call and was assured an ambulance would be sent shortly to pick her up. I stayed with the girl and her extremely distraught parents and never left their sides until the ambulance arrived. I felt I was not only rendering treatment but providing a presence and even a shoulder for the parents to weep on. After all, they were my patients too.

Cybil had a prolonged stay at the other hospital after the required exchange transfusion. Fortunately her liver and kidney function remained normal as the rapid intervention of treatment of the elevated acetaminophen level apparently prevented their damage. Upon discharge, arrangements were made for her to be under the care of a psychiatrist, and she and the family followed up with this diligently. In view of the unusual situation of both daughters in the same family making a serious suicide attempt, the Division of Youth and Family Services was also contacted to make their assessment of the family dynamics.

Although I was not involved in their psychiatric care, I did see both daughters on occasion in my office for minor ailments. They were always attractively groomed and were cheerful and seemed happy. I never really understood what caused them each to make such a serious suicide attempt which nearly cost them their lives.

Suicide is the second leading cause of death among teen-agers in the United States. The most frequent causes were jumping from high places and overdosing on pills. Jumping from high places was easy for me to understand as on several occasions I had to stop my own sons from doing that. On one occasion my older son attempted that after fashioning a cape from a large towel, which he assumed that, since it seemed to protect Superman, it would do the same for him. Fortunately, my husband and I intervened in time. Children watch a lot of those cartoon heroes doing all sorts of super feats, and they assume they should be able to do them too.

However, overdosing on pills is a lot harder to under-stand. In recent years there has been a huge increase in the frequency of teen suicides. People who have studied the problem have attributed this to bullying, especially cyber-bullying which occurs more often now with the rise in the availability and use of smart phones. It has been estimated that the average amount of smart phone usage by teens is about five hours a day. It has also been shown that those teens who are glued to their smart phones that long are 70 percent more likely to have suicidal thoughts. Excessive smart phone usage can also lead to sleep deprivation, poor school performance, and absenteeism. Social media can also add to the stress on teenagers by increasing their need to keep up appearances and to perform beyond their natural abilities. Added to all this is the stress of prepping for college admittance and overscheduling of activities so as to have a more impressive resume.

Not being privy to the innermost thoughts or behavior of the Barone daughters, I never really knew what caused their suicide attempts. I continued to see them for a number of years afterward and was happy that they made no further attempts, as it is said that if someone really wants to commit suicide they really cannot be stopped.

One day I got a request from the older daughter to perform a premarital physical for her and her fiancé. I was happy to oblige and sent them both off with my very best wishes. The younger daughter, who was an extraordinary athlete, came in not long after for a physical needed for the college which had awarded her a full scholarship and which she was about to enter. I performed this for her and sent her off with a warm hug.

I continued to see the parents until my own retirement. Since I continued to live in the same community I would often see my patients at the supermarket or the mall. I have seen the Barones now and then and am always happy to receive their delighted reports on how everything is going in the lives of their lovely daughters. The older girl, I was told proudly, had recently made them grandparents. When I left them, I had to suppress my tears of joy at hearing this wonderful news.

Brandon

❧❧

For many of the thirty-five years that I have spent practicing medicine, I was the only female General Practitioner in the area. When I went to medical school, female medical students were few and far between, and most of them went into either pediatrics or psychiatry. Our presence was often resented by the male medical students and residents, and they often made life very unpleasant for us. To make life even more difficult, special provisions such as female changing rooms and female on-call rooms were not made available for us. I recall one day when we asked where we should "gown up," we were told to go in with the nurses. Several of us resented that there were no accommodations for us as there were for the male students, and so we went in and changed in the doctor's lounge with all the male students. This created quite a stir but at least our point was made. I will not chronicle all the embarrassments and humiliations that we were subject to. That would take an entire other book. I do recall having to physically restrain my husband one day from going up on the hospital floor and punching out one of the residents who treated me very badly. My husband kept insisting that he had no right to treat me so disrespectfully, but although I agreed, I impressed upon him that it would only make things worse for me. I am happy to see that things have changed considerably with many more females entering the medical profession and the accompanying acceptance of their presence.

When I opened my practice in a suburban area of NJ, there was only one female pediatrician and no female Family Practitioners in the area. However, since there were really not enough primary care doctors to serve the area, my office was flooded from day one. My patients came from a large catchment area, but interestingly nearly all were females and children. Rarely did I ever see the husbands or fathers in the early years of my practice. Often the only times I would ever get to meet the husbands was when they had to accompany their wives or mothers to the office, the emergency room, or the hospital. Many patients came afterward on referral from friends or family, and some just picked my name out of the phone book because they preferred to have a female physician. For that reason, I did a lot of office gynecology with some patients coming from distances more than two hours away. There is a large population of women who would die sooner than go to a male physician for an intimate exam, and soon after opening my office I saw women with serious gynecologic problems who had not seen a physician for more than twenty years. I recall one woman coming in with a cancerous growth about the size of a lemon who had refused to see a male physician for the problem. It took a great deal of persuasion to get her to agree to see a male surgeon, as there were no female surgeons for many miles around and she needed urgent care. I even offered to go with her and hold her hand, but she gratefully declined my offer.

Most patients would come into the office for legitimate reasons, but every now and then I was the victim of kooks, drug seekers, and perverts. So, when a new male patient called one day to seek an appointment for a problem involving his genitals, a mini alarm went off in my mind.

On the day of his appointment we had a busy office schedule and I forgot about his arrival. When he arrived, the nurse had him fill out the usual forms and then placed him in the examination room and told him I would be coming in shortly. It is my custom never to have people undress before they meet with me. I think there is something humiliating and embarrassing for a patient to be sitting up on the examination table in a dressing gown which barely covers their nakedness while they are meeting someone for the first time. So, when I entered the room and found the patient standing stark naked looking out the window I was quite shocked. No one had told him to undress. I quickly threw a drape at him and asked him to sit down and cover himself while I left the room again to regain my composure.

When I came back in, the patient told me he was having a lot of pain in his genital area. I questioned him about what he thought might be the cause of this and if he had ever had this problem before. He said he had never had it before and had no idea what caused it. Since my examination did not reveal any objective findings, I just recommended some innocuous conservative measures to deal with his complaint. When he left, he made an appointment for follow-up the next week even though I told him he only needed to come back if the problem did not improve. Also, he did not pay his bill. Certain that he was just another thrill-seeking patient, I checked his registration form on which he claimed to have been referred by an orthopedic surgeon in the area.

By that evening I had forgotten the incident and attended a staff Christmas party at the hospital. When I saw the orthopedic surgeon that the patient had named on his registration form, it prodded my memory, and since it was general seating, I sat down next to him so I could ask him about the patient. I asked him if he recalled referring the patient to my office. He could not remember doing so but said he would check the patient's chart and get back to me.

The week passed uneventfully, and the day of the patient's appointment arrived. So certain was I that he would not return that we booked another patient in his time slot. However, he did arrive at the designated time and professed no end of gratitude for my suggestions and the improvement in his medical condition. And, on the way out, he paid the bill for both visits.

Later that afternoon, the specialist called me to say that he had checked the chart and that the young man was indeed his patient and yes, he had referred him to me during a recent visit because the man said he had a female physician where he lived before and would like to sign up with one again in his new location.

I was certainly glad that, despite my overwhelming suspicions, I had given him the benefit of the doubt and treated him as I would any other patient.

During thirty-five years of medical practice I saw many different illnesses and many different reactions to illness. The reactions ranged from sadness, fear, anger, blame, and surprisingly, even pleasure. To treat these people effectively I needed to be cognizant of these reactions. My staff would often comment to me that so and so was acting "funny" and even displaying anger, belligerence, and rudeness to them. I had to remind them that if they were not sick, they would not be coming here, and it was our responsibility to care them and not them to care for us.

In Brandon's case, although suspecting at first he was not here for a legitimate reason, I treated him as if he were and it turned out he was. He remained in my care for many years afterward.

Louise

ఆఅఅఅ

Louise was an African American woman who had been in my practice for about the last ten years. My practice was in a bedroom community of New York City and was composed mainly of white and blue collar workers. It was the type of community that was often referred to as "Middle America". In the early years of my practice there, there were very few African Americans that lived in the community and so did not compose much of my practice. However, with the advent of Managed Care with many patients receiving the medical care provided by their employment, people came to us from communities that were further away. Louise was an example of that.

Louise was a woman in her late sixties who had had an unsuccessful marriage early in her life and had raised a lovely daughter by herself. She was an executive secretary, and her daughter was employed as a nursing supervisor. I usually saw Louise only about once or twice a year for minor ailments. Often when brought into the examination room she would apologize to me for taking up my time with her trivial complaints. I tried to tell her that if her complaints mattered to her, they mattered to me.

One day however, as I was bustling from room to room my nurse stopped me in the hallway to warn me that Louise was in one of the examination rooms and to be prepared to see an extremely distressed lady.

As I entered the room, I was immediately aware of two things. One was that Louise was in fact extremely distressed with a tear-streaked face and audibly sobbing, and the second was the cause of her distress. Louise had pale patches all over her face and arms. I knew immediately that she was suffering from Vitiligo which, although quite harmless, was obviously very distressing to her. She began to ask me why this had happened to her, and I said that the cause was unknown while at the same time reassuring her that it was not dangerous or life-threatening in any way, but also that it would probably progress. She said she already knew this, but it seemed to offer her little solace. I asked her to tell me why it was so distressing to her as it was not at all painful and I didn't think it was the cosmetic effect that was particularly bothering her.

She hesitated a few moments before answering. She then said that she was quite adjusted to being a black woman and was happy with that but that now she felt she was no longer black and not white either. She felt that she didn't know where she fit. She said, "What am I now, Dr. Robertson?"

I didn't really have an answer for her, so I focused on re-assuring her that it would have no effect on her health and that all she had to be careful about was exposure to the sun. I explained that the pale patches on her skin represented a loss of the pigment melanin which is nature's best sunscreen and those areas could be easily burned by sun exposure and that she should cover up and use sunscreen when outdoors. But I also told her that the disease was progressive—in some people rapidly progressive and in others slowly progressive. I suspected it would be rapidly progressive in her case as she already had large pale areas which had developed in a rel-atively short time.

Louise left the office, and I didn't see her for close to another year. This time when I entered the examination room, Louise was all smiles. I was immediately struck when I noticed that the previously noted pale patches on her face were becoming pigmented again and were much less notice-able. She then showed me her arms, and the pale patches were almost entirely gone. I asked her what she had done to make this happen, and she said it was the power of prayer. She said she prayed every night and asked God to make her an all-black lady again, and she said He was answering her prayers. I was flabbergasted as I had never known a case of vitiligo to regress, but I also learned never to argue with success or the methods used to achieve it.

During many years of medical practice, I had learned that it was important to learn people's belief systems and to work with them rather than against them. Belief systems can be very powerful, and in order to be an effective physician for my patients, it served both them and myself better to work with them rather than against them. Louise firmly believed that her prayers caused her disease to regress and who was I, a confirmed agnostic, to argue with her? So, I took her hands in mine, and we prayed together that day for her disease to continue to regress and never come back. And if Louise was smiling before I came into the room, she was now smiling from ear to ear upon leaving.

Managed care patients were often shifted from one plan to another as employers sought to control costs and went with the plan that offered the best prices that week. So Louise and her daughter were lost, along with many others, to my practice, while others came in from new employers. However, she did call in from time to time and reported that although her illness didn't get completely better, it had not gotten any worse and was much better than when I originally saw her. I was happy to hear this but wistful at not seeing her and her daughter anymore. She was an especially delightful lady, always polite, respectful, and beautifully groomed.

That doesn't necessarily describe all the patients coming to the office. Illness often impacts negatively on people's behaviors, and it was not infrequent that my staff would complain to me about their rudeness. I always had the same answer. I told them that if they were not sick, they would not be here, and it was our job to take care of them and not their job to take care of us. When ill, many people are so tuned into themselves, their pain, and their discomfort that they lose sight of their surroundings and the people around them.

I lived close to my office and so would often see patients in the supermarket or the mall nearby. It never ceased to amaze me that when I said "hello" to them they would look at me quizzically as if to say, "Gee you look familiar to me but I can't quite place you or know who you are." However, if they had a child with them, the child would immediately recognize me and say, "Oh, there's Dr. Robertson."

Lucy

❧

I had a sizeable Medicaid practice because while many primary care practices in the area had quotas on the number they would accept, we had none.

Lucy had been a patient of mine for about five years. I knew she lived alone in a local boarding house. She was twenty-five years old when I first met with her, and I saw her only once or twice a year for minor ailments.

Lucy was a warm, friendly lady, but was quite unattractive. She had a badly pockmarked face, the residue of untreated teenage acne, small eyes, and a hooked nose. In addition she had a bad case of scoliosis which also should have been recognized in adolescence but was not treated. She had never completed high school, having to go out at an early age and earn a living. All in all, she was a rather unattractive and unhappy woman. I learned that she supported herself by cleaning houses and had recently acquired jobs to clean offices and buildings as well.

One visit she came and reported to me that she had met a man that she liked and that they were dating. His name was Mike and he worked as a janitor at one of the buildings in which she cleaned. He was about ten years older than her but had never married. In fact, she said he had never dated.

About a month later they called the office to report that they were planning to marry and needed their premarital physicals and blood work to get their license. When they appeared at the office, Lucy was all smiles and so was Mike, and I couldn't help noticing that half of his teeth were missing. They both seemed very happy and devoted to each other, and I was happy for them.

They rented an apartment nearby, and I continued to see Lucy now and then for minor ailments. However, each time she came in, she lamented to me that she wished she could get pregnant as they both so much wanted a child and to start a family. During one visit, after they had been married for three years, she came in sobbing because she couldn't get pregnant and asked me what she could do. She feared that because she was now thirty-four years old, she would never be able to get pregnant. I knew they could never afford the services of a Fertility Physician with the attendant expensive workup and testing, so I just suggested to her some simple techniques that might increase the likeliness of her conceiving. I told her to put one or two pillows under her bum during intercourse, and to remain in that position for a while afterward. Also, I cautioned her to remain in bed and not to get up for the rest of the night.

About six months later, Lucy came once again into the office, but this time to report that she had missed her menses for the last two months. She looked imploringly at me to do a pregnancy test for her, as she knew this was not reimbursable under Medicaid. This was in the day when the tests could only be done in a lab or a doctor's office, as they were not yet available in pharmacies. Lucy waited for the result in one of the examination rooms, and when I came back in to report that the test was positive and that she was indeed pregnant, she jumped up and hugged me. We both did a little victory dance and then the office staff came in and joined in the festivities.

I referred Lucy to one of the local obstetricians who accepted Medicaid patients for her maternity care as, because of her age, she was considered high risk for a problematic pregnancy.

About seven months later, I received a call from the hospital that she had delivered a baby boy and that all had gone well with the delivery, and that the baby was doing fine. Since they had chosen me to do his infant care, I went to the hospital shortly after to see them and examine the new baby.

Upon arrival at the Newborn Nursery, the nurse informed me that the baby was in the room with the new parents. When I walked into the room, Lucy was reclining in the bed and the husband was seated in a chair nearby, looking down at the baby he was holding in his arms. He was positioned in front of a window with bright sunlight streaming in which silhouetted him and created a halo of light around him. The scene was so beautiful it looked to me like a religious painting done by Raphael or Caravaggio. Their shared happiness also seemed to create a glow in the room which struck me as something like a divine religious experience. That moment of extreme joy and beauty I experienced in that room is one I can never forget.

I continued to see them and their son, whom they also named Mike after the father, for many years later unto his teens. They did not have any more children and totally doted on little Mike. Mike was a cheerful, affable boy and didn't seem to be spoiled by all the love and attention his parents devoted on him. After I retired from my work, Lucy remained in contact with me periodically as I often gave my home number to my patients.

At first when I did this, other doctors warned me that I would be hounded by patients at all hours of the day and night, but that never happened. I never had a single patient abuse that privilege. I felt that it was especially necessary for new parents to know that help was readily available as so many felt so insecure in their new role.

Unfortunately, Mike the father died when little Mike was in his teens. The father was a labile diabetic, a disease which was difficult to control, and he slipped one night into a diabetic coma. Lucy and little Mike were devastated when I saw them at the funeral. However, they supported each other, and not long after, Lucy was offered a job as a caretaker in a large gracious home in south Jersey. The job came with a small residence on the property and so she and little Mike moved there. Lucy remained in contact with me for a long time thereafter.

I'll never know whether the suggestions I made to Lucy were what led to her pregnancy, but that didn't daunt the joy and happiness I had from being able to share with them the pleasure they always had having little Mike as their son.

I've had other patients that had difficulties in conceiving. Their care under Fertility Physicians not uncommonly went into the hundreds of thousands of dollars and, even then, was not always successful. Oftentimes the problem was created by couples waiting too long to start a family. Despite my warning that fertility significantly declines after age thirty, they felt it was more important for them to delay starting a family and keep working so they could afford the upkeep of a new home, or two cars, or expensive vacations. Too often they paid a heavy price for those luxuries.

Arthur

❧✦❧

Arthur's mother, Claudia, started suddenly to have significant bleeding at the twentieth week of her pregnancy. Everything had gone smoothly with her pregnancy, but her prenatal care had been sporadic because her husband was with the armed services and had been recently stationed at several different bases. Since she was thirty-five years old, under more normal circumstances her pregnancy would have been followed with an ultrasound to rule out Down's syndrome or other prenatal difficulties, but that had not been done. Upon presentation to the emergency room at the start of the bleeding, it was determined that her hemoglobin level had dropped enough to admit her to the hospital and transfuse her with several units of blood. Ultrasound revealed she had a condition called placenta previa which is the abnormal placement of the placenta in the uterus. Usually the placenta is attached to the uterus high up but in about one out of one hundred pregnancies, it attaches partially or completely over the cervix. As the pregnancy continues, the cervix begins to thin out to prepare the uterus for childbirth, and the integrity of the abnormal placental attachment becomes compromised and bleeding often ensues.

Claudia's condition was considered serious, so it was decided to keep Claudia in the hospital for observation, so that immediate treatment could be given should she start to bleed again. She did well for a number of weeks but at week thirty-three she had another massive bleed and an immediate C section had to be performed. She delivered an infant boy who weighed about one and a half pounds at birth and had an Apgar score of 1.

The Apgar score was named for Virginia Apgar, who, in 1952 devised the score as a means of assessing a baby's status at one minute and five minutes after birth. It is a means of quickly summarizing the health of a newborn and determines the amount of immediate care and attention required.

The score evaluates the heart rate, color, muscle tone, respiration, and response to stimuli. Each aspect is measured on a scale of 0 to 2, 0 being absent and 2 being good, as expected.

Arthur's Apgar score at one minute was 1, based on a slow heart rate—less than 100 beats per minute. He was a zero on all the other factors and he was cyanotic, flaccid, unresponsive, and not breathing. He exhibited no cry. At five minutes, the Apgar score had increased to 2, as with immediate mouth to mouth resuscitation that was administered, his color had somewhat improved. He was placed in an incubator on a ventilator and brought to the Neonatal Intensive Care Unit.

An infant's lungs do not become mature until at about thirty-six weeks of pregnancy. Immature lungs do not have a sufficient amount of a substance called surfactant which keeps the air sacs from sticking together and enables them to stay open. Unless they are open, they cannot accomplish taking in oxygen and giving off carbon dioxide appropriately. Then the infant does not receive enough oxygen and develops a condition called Neonatal Respiratory Distress Syndrome.

Artificial surfactant was administered almost immediately, and the infant had a modest improvement in color. However the ventilator had to be continued for a number of weeks to do the breathing for the infant and provide high levels of oxygen.

The distraught parents were notified of the infant's condition and told that he would have to be kept in the Neonatal ICU for the time being. The parents gave the name "Arthur" to the baby and begged the staff to do everything to save him. They had no other children, and Claudia had had a very difficult time getting pregnant in the first place. The time turned out to be four months, during which Claudia came every day to the ICU. She pumped her breast milk and brought it and fed it to him with a medicine dropper as she held him.

After four months, Arthur had gained enough weight to considered for discharge and was able to take in foods. He seemed to be able to recognize his mother and even started to smile when she arrived. However, it was apparent to the staff and the parents that he was nevertheless severely handicapped as he showed no signs of being able to move his arms or legs.

I first saw Arthur when he was about five years old. The parents had just recently moved into our neighborhood and approached me to do the medical care of the family. The mother carried Arthur into the office and then the examination room as he was never able to walk. She brought him in that day for me to meet them and become aware of his condition. I performed a physical examination and didn't find any significant problems at that time except for making notes on his severe physical handicap which was evidenced by the extreme atrophy noted in both his arms and legs. Arthur was able to sit up on the examination table, but only with some support from his mother, but he was barely able to lift his head. I chatted with him, and he seemed to be quite aware and even displayed a sense of humor making some funny remarks to me about the other children and toys in the waiting room. Claudia had brought along his medical records which I checked to assure them that all his shots were up to date. She also presented a bulging folder with his records from birth, which, because of a busy office schedule, I asked her to leave with me so I could peruse them at my leisure. That evening I sat down to read the records which is how I learned about all that happened during Claudia's pregnancy and Arthur's stay in the NICU which stands for Neonatal Intensive Care Unit.

I would see Arthur about every few months for minor illnesses, and Claudia always had to carry him into the office. He seemed cheerful enough and always gave me a friendly "hi Doc".

One day, Arthur's mother called for an appointment, saying Arthur was sick. She brought him in later that morning, and the nurse informed me after she admitted him that he had a temperature of 102 degrees. When I came in to see him, Claudia began to tell me that he started to complain of a sore throat the evening before and even asked her to bring him to me. Arthur looked pretty washed out sitting there on the examination table as his mother supported him. He was still unable to lift his head but his eyes peered at me past the lowered head. And suddenly, he interrupted his mother as she gave me his history and said, "Let ME tell her, Mommy."

When he said that, I felt as if I had been struck with a beam. Tears came to my eyes as I realized that this little boy who really had nothing—no mobility, no future, no hope of ever improving—had suddenly struggled to assert the only thing he had left, his personhood. I said, "Of course, Arthur," and patiently listened as he took up where his mother left off. After that whenever I saw Arthur I made it my business to converse mostly with him and always take the time to listen patiently.

However, about a year later, my secretary informed me that Arthur's mother had called to tell us that she could no longer bring Arthur to our office and asked if we would please forward his records to another doctor. I called her back after office hours were finished, and she thanked me profusely for the time and loving care I rendered to Arthur but explained that he was getting too heavy for her to carry him up all the steps to my office. I said that I understood but to know that I will always be there for them in any way in which they should need me.

As I lived in a community near my office, it was not infrequent that I would run into my patients at the mall or the supermarket. About a year later, I did run into Claudia and Arthur who was being wheeled in a stroller, and Arthur gave me a bright enthusiastic greeting and even told me he liked me better than his new doctor. I told him that since I was no longer his doctor, it would be okay for me to give him a kiss—which I did. And he blushed so becomingly when I did that.

I can never forget that very moving moment in the office when Arthur said, "Let ME tell her, Mommy." Tears come to my eyes every time I recall it.

Julie

࿂࿂࿂

I'd known Julie since birth as her parents had been patients of mine for many years, and when her mother became pregnant with her, they asked me to do her infant and ongoing care.

Her early years were uncomplicated. She was a charming and delightful and easy to care for baby, and so after the immunization schedule was completed, I only saw her occasionally for minor illnesses.

In high school she was an avid track participant, and so I would see her more often during this time for her yearly school physicals which were required for athletic participation. At first she specialized in short distance runs but then decided she preferred to do long distance runs. Despite being offered several college scholarships upon graduation from high school, she decided to take time off to train to run marathons. She ran several local marathons and qualified to run the Boston Marathon.

After a while she decided she didn't want to go to college and opened up a sporting goods store in a neighboring town. The store was successful and was finally bought out by a major sporting goods store.

At one of these marathons she met another runner, and they started dating and fell in love. They became engaged and one day presented in my office requesting their premarital physicals and blood work. They came in on a Friday and told me the wedding was planned for a week from the following Saturday. It was to be held in a church in their town to be followed by a huge reception afterward as they both had many friends and large extended families. Since all preparations had been completed, Julie and her fiancé Tom had decided to go on an outreach program the following week as they both loved the outdoors and figured it would be a good way to escape all the pre-wedding jitters.

Everything went well with their premarital physicals, and they were both found to be in excellent health. Blood was drawn for VDRL studies. VDRL stands for Venereal Disease Research Laboratory test and screens for antibodies for exposure to syphilis. It is a required test to obtain a marriage license.

I wished them well on their outreach program and assured them that the results would be waiting for them upon their return so they could then go and get the marriage license.

Several days later the lab results came back, but since we had such a busy office schedule, I didn't open them until the end of office hours that day. When I did open them, I was stunned to see that Julie's test came back positive. I knew this was not a terribly uncommon happening and did not signal that Julie had or had been exposed to syphilis. However, I also knew that would be reason enough to deny the issuance of their marriage license. With all the marriage preparations in place, it would be a catastrophe if the wedding had to be delayed.

I called her parents' home and told them I needed to see Julie and Tom as soon as possible. Her mother told me that they were not expected to return until either late Thursday or early Friday. I impressed upon her the urgency of them contacting me as soon as they arrived.

Late Thursday evening, my answering service called me to tell me that a young lady had been calling franticly and said it was extremely urgent to reach me. I called back and arranged to see both Julie and Tom first thing the next morning. Although I had a hospital meeting to attend, I skipped it and met with them both in my office.

They were shocked when I told them that Julie's screening test for syphilis had come back positive. I immediately explained that it was not the most sensitive test and that now and then false positives occurred. In that event it was necessary to send another test which was much more specific for the detection of syphilis. When they asked me why that test wasn't done in the first place, I explained that it was a more expensive test to perform and that the VDRL is sufficient for screening in most cases. I assured both of them of the unlikeliness of the more specific test also coming back positive. The only problem now was how to get the result back in time so they could acquire their marriage license. This was the Friday before the wedding which was to take place the next day. They had to get the license that day so that the marriage could go through the following day.

I knew if I just drew the blood for the more specific test and waited for the normal turnaround time, the result would not be available until the following week. So after drawing the blood, I drove down to the lab which did the analysis and begged the people to do the test right then and there. They were reluctant to gratify my request but when I explained the reason for the urgency, they finally agreed to do it. As expected, the test came back negative. I hurriedly returned to my office and gave Julie and Tom the paper confirming the negative results and they ran off to the Town Hall and got the marriage license without further event.

Julie became pregnant in less than a year after marriage and then had three more children in the next five years. She still runs marathons but smaller ones. I see her and the children quite frequently for routine infant care, and we laugh together each time reminiscing about how their marriage almost needed to be cancelled.

Julie and Tom are now grandparents. Since we live in the same town, I see them and their children and new grandchild now and then. I do not do their medical care any longer as I have been retired from my medical practice several years hence. However, as we all still live in the same town, I see them frequently on walks, or on visits to the supermarket or mall. We still smile and laugh together remembering the traumatic day before their wedding.

Melissa

୧⌒୨

My first position after completing my Family Practice Residency was in a Family Practice clinic headed by an immensely popular physician fondly called "Dr. Tom" by his patients. I was mystified by his popularity because there were several other Family Practice clinics in the area, yet they were not as well liked or attended. Indeed, many days I had to weave my way through the front door because it was blocked by patients spilling over from the waiting room, which was already filled to capacity. Parking within a several block radius was impossible because the streets were filled with his waiting patients, many arriving in the early morning before the clinic opened.

One morning I awoke with a painful stiff neck and shoulder. By the time I got to the clinic, I was carrying my head at an awkward angle, obviously in considerable pain. Dr. Tom immediately noticed this. Before I could protest, he came up swiftly behind me and placed his large hands on my neck and shoulders. I immediately became aware of a feeling of warmth, comfort, and relaxation. I smiled, the pain seemed to lessen, and I knew I would be better soon. Dr. Tom was a master of the art of "laying on of the hands".

This incident was to have considerable influence on my own practice of medicine through the years. I was liberal in my use of touch and frequently held my patient's hands or placed my hands to rest on painful areas for a few seconds before performing my examination. The patient was comforted, and the relaxation enabled me to perform a better physical examination without the involuntary guarding physicians usually encounter.

Melissa's mother had been my patient for a number of years, but I had never met her daughter because she lived out of town. However, I learned from her mother that she had recently fallen on hard times and that she was once again living with her mother.

One day Melissa called the office to have sutures removed from her scalp. Apparently she had taken a bad fall and had gone to the ER of the local hospital where a deep scalp wound had been sutured. She was then told to follow up with her family physician to have the sutures removed after ten days.

She was brought into the examination room where the nurse cleansed the wound in preparation for the suture removal. I entered soon after and immediately noticed and commented on the strong resemblance she had to her mother.

I then repositioned her on a chair in the room because she was a tall girl and too high for me to reach while seated on the examination table. It was a habit of my practice to place my hands for a moment or two on my patient so they could get accustomed to their presence and then relax. This is particularly effective in performing an abdominal examination because when the muscles are relaxed I am able to palpate the internal organs much more effectively. So, with Melissa positioned comfortably on a chair, I stood behind her and placed my hands on her scalp. I immediately noticed a very strange sensation. I felt that there was a vibration when I touched her scalp. I removed my hands and turned around and faced her and asked if she was very nervous about what I was about to do. She responded that she wasn't nervous at all, that she was a tomboy growing up, and that she had had sutures removed a number of times before. I returned to my position behind her head and once again placed my hands on her scalp. I still noticed the strange sensation of a vibration, which made me think of something that had been plugged into an electrical socket. Once again I turned to face her and asked her to hold her arms out in front of her. When she did that, I noticed that there was a fine tremor present. That made me realize a more thorough examination was in order, so I took her pulse, temperature, and blood pressure. Both pulse and heart rate were found to be significantly elevated, and she had an oral temperature of 101.5 degrees Fahrenheit. Further examination of her neck revealed a bruit or whooshing noise over her thyroid gland. I also noticed now a mild swelling over her neck which without the other findings might easily have been missed since she was a rather chubby girl.

I informed her that some blood studies needed to be done which she immediately refused to do. She told me she was starting a new job the next week and that her insurance with the new company would not kick in for another month. She said she would return at that time for the blood studies but could not do them now as she could not pay for them. I told her they needed to be done now and that she could pay me whenever she could, even in small increments if that was all she could manage. This took quite a bit of convincing, but she finally agreed.

I drew the blood and sent it off requesting a stat (to be done immediately) result. After I removed the sutures without event, Melissa left the office, and I promised her I would let her know the results as soon as they were available.

That evening the lab called me to tell me that her thyroid function studies were the most elevated they had ever seen in the lab. I realized this signaled a possible impending thyroid storm which is a potentially life-threatening event. This is a condition where an individual's heart rate, blood pressure, and body temperature can soar to such dangerously high levels that it could cause death. The condition is usually caused by an illness or extreme stress in an individual. I suspected in Melissa's case there might have been a significant stress in her life which caused her to suddenly move back to live with her mother. It also might have been brought on by whatever trauma she underwent when she sustained the laceration on her scalp which required the sutures. A number of conditions can cause thyroid storm, even something like a punch in the throat. But the cause was not what was important right now. She needed immediate treatment with thyroid suppressant medications and beta blockers to control heart rate and blood pressure.

I telephoned her mother's house to deliver the results but received no answer. Knowing that Melissa's treatment couldn't be delayed, I went to their house but found them not to be at home. I knocked on the door of a neighbor's apartment and asked if she knew of their whereabouts. She said they had spoken earlier of taking in a movie that evening, and that they should be back home soon. So I waited and shortly thereafter they appeared. Since it was already late in the evening and I knew all pharmacies would be closed, I told Melissa she needed to be admitted to the hospital for immediate treatment. This again brought vehement objections because of her uninsured status, but when I explained the condition was very serious and could be life-threatening (which my presence at their house late in the evening underscored), her mother said she would assume all financial responsibility for her, and she was promptly admitted to the hospital. She was treated for the next few days with medications to stabilize her condition and was discharged feeling a lot better.

Upon discharge I referred her to an endocrinologist for management, and she was treated with radioactive iodine and did well. A few days later her mother came to my office and paid the bill for her lab tests, saying she preferred that her daughter should owe her the money rather than me.

I continued to see Melissa for a number of years after until she married and moved to another area. Her mother tells me that Melissa has made her a grandmother and is doing well.

The tradition of the laying on of the hands originated in the Old Testament of the Bible and is also mentioned in the New Testament. It is accorded to be a means of blessing or praying for healing. The practice of it certainly worked in this event.

Peter

❧◉◎☙

The area that I practiced in had until recently been a rural farm area. The main highway leading out from the city had ended about five miles before our town. However, when that stretch of highway finally got completed, our rural community soon got transformed into a bedroom community of the big city. What followed soon after was the purchase of large tracts of land by developers and the construction of high priced housing. And soon, following on the heels of the sudden availability of new homes, was the influx of doctors to serve the new residents. However, before that all happened, I opened my Family Practice and was inundated with appointment requests by the first day as there were very few Family Doctors in the area and even fewer specialists. I found myself performing a lot of tasks in my office that were new to me as I had formerly practiced in the big city where there were many specialists available to call upon.

However, one day I needed to refer a patient for a gynecologic procedure and sent her to Peter, the only Ob Gyn guy that was in our town. I had met him a number of times in the hospital lounge, and he never even greeted me whereas most of the other physicians welcomed me to the staff. I also knew he didn't have the most pleasant bedside manner, but since he was the only act in town, I referred my patient to him.

About a week or so later the patient came back to my office, and when I asked her how the procedure went, she said she was in the operating room but was so put off by the manner of the gynecologist that she got off the table and told him to "go fly a kite" and that she wasn't going to let him touch her. I was shocked to hear this but told her that she still needed the procedure, and so I referred her to another person who was quite far away and worked in a different hospital.

Fortunately, more doctors soon came into our area, and I did not need to refer to Peter anymore.

Sometime later I learned that his wife was expecting their third child. The first two children were girls, and Peter was loudly hoping for a boy. We had a party every year at the hospital which was called an "Ice Breaker" which was held to welcome new doctors and their spouses to the staff. I met his wife Margaret at the party and we sat together and chatted for a while. Margaret was past thirty-five at the time and would have been recommended to have an amniocentesis to check for any possibility of fetal abnormalities, but she declined the procedure because she was a staunch Catholic and told me that she would not terminate the pregnancy no matter what was found. She was then in her seventh month and feeling well.

About two months later I was walking down the hall of the hospital where I was on staff, and noticed a noisy gathering at the end of the hall. I could tell that Peter seemed to be at the center of it, but didn't know what it was all about. I later learned that his wife had delivered that morning, and that the baby, a boy, had Down's syndrome. Peter, of course did not deliver the baby, and was nearby at the birth, but stormed off raging when he saw the child. He totally rejected the child and would visit his wife only when the child was not with her. She was devastated by all this but remained firm in her decision to keep and care for the baby.

She chose me to do the newborn infant care for the child, first at the hospital and then followed up in my office. This was against Peter's advice as he was disturbed at my not referring patients to him for quite a while. At every visit she cried and told me that Peter still would have nothing to do with the baby.

The baby was in good health, tolerated all the shots well, and after the first six months, I did not see Margaret and the baby for another six months. They did come in for the one year checkup and Margaret reported that Peter seemed to be softening in his approach to the child. He would pick him up now and then when he was crying and even once offered to feed him when Margaret was busy with the other children. Down's syndrome children are so cheerful and full of smiles they are hard to resist. I was delighted to learn that Peter seemed to be accepting the child. The other girls and Margaret showered attention on the baby boy, and he was acquiring all the milestones in an acceptable manner. There is a spectrum of the Down's handicap and the boy, whom they named Matthew, seemed to have a rather mild case.

As the years went by, I saw Margaret and Matthew at their regular visits, and each time Margaret reported the good news that Peter was now treating Matthew just as a regular member of their family, and even taking delight in his cheeriness. He was spending time with him and trying to teach him new skills.

I would run into Peter at the hospital, usually in the doctor's lounge, and he was friendly and sociable and seemed to be a different person. I decided to risk referring a patient to him and the lady came back to me with a happy report of the care she had received.

I asked myself, what seemed to cause this radical transformation? I don't have any certain answers to this, but I suspect the suffering Peter endured by having a less than perfect child, made him more sensitive and attuned to the suffering of others, and therefore a more effective physician and decent human being.

Brian

❧⦿❧

Brian was born to a forty-four-year-old mother. When I have been asked to do the care of the infant, I am not usually in the delivery room at the birth, but I get called shortly afterward. However, when the pregnancy is considered high risk as in this case—an infant born to an elderly mother, — the presence of a physician to care for the infant is requested. Another situation in which the physician for the infant is requested is in what is commonly called "the precious child syndrome". This is a child born to parents who have lost children either at birth or afterward, or the parents are very unlikely to ever have another child.

Brian was what is often referred to as "a change of life baby". The mother had previously delivered five daughters, the oldest being twenty-four and the youngest being twelve.

So when she realized that she was once again pregnant, it came as a shock to her and the entire family. However, when ultrasound revealed that the fetus was a male, everyone was very happy after having had five daughters, and they eagerly anticipated the birth.

Everything went smoothly with the pregnancy, and the delivery was rapid and uncomplicated. The infant was full sized, weighed seven pounds, eight ounces, and had an excellent Apgar score. Everyone breathed a sigh of relief. However, I immediately noticed that the infant was what we refer to as a "funny looking baby". There are whole books written about this phenomenon with photos and descriptions of associated anomalies which often go along with the odd looking face. I noticed that Brian, who had been named before he was even born, had an unusually large head and close set eyes. Often these syndromes are caused by a genetic anomaly, which because all the other daughters seemed not to have a similar look, I suspected might have been due either to a mutation or possibly a Y chromosome-linked anomaly which of course would not have affected the girls.

After Brian was cleaned up and brought to the newborn nursery, I performed a thorough examination but did not find any associated anomalies. Usually infants having the "funny looking child syndrome" have other associated anomalies. Brian did not appear to have any. I went out to the lounge where the father and all five daughters eagerly awaited the news and told them that everything went well with the delivery and Brian was in good health. I did not mention his "funny look" at this time because I wanted to research the subject and be more certain of my findings. They were all so ecstatic at now having a boy in the family, I didn't feel I wanted to unduly alarm everyone before I was certain of my suspicions.

That evening I sat down with one of the "funny looking kids" books but didn't quite find any syndrome that fit my findings. I called one of the other pediatricians and asked him to look in on Brian when he visited the nursery and tell me his impression of Brian's facial appearance. We talked again the next day and he said he also noted the large head and close set eyes, but too was unable to fit his look into any of the known syndromes. He concluded, "Look, he just might be a funny looking kid, and that's that."

I continued to see Brian for his regularly scheduled infant visits and was pleased at how well he was thriving. Often the visits were accompanied not only by the mother but also by at least several of the daughters. They were all obviously smitten with the baby and doted on him. The mother said that his father, upon returning from work every day, could barely take off his coat before going into Brian's room to pick him up and play with him.

Brian attained all the milestones, crawling, walking and talking at the usual times. Since his development was so normal, I discarded my original concern about Brian having one of the "funny looking kid" syndromes. However, at each visit I could not help but notice the excessive care and attention he was receiving from the family members. They watched, hovered, and protected him at every turn and in effect were rendering him pretty helpless. They kept him at home and didn't allow him to play with other children, lest, as they told me, they hurt him or transmit an illness to him. When he started kindergarten, he hardly ever attended as the parents seemed to find any and every excuse to keep him home. I had the feeling that they were treating him as a precious doll to be protected at any and every turn.

This treatment of Brian continued despite my many comments that it could be affecting his development. As time went on, Brian became more and more dependent on the family members doing everything for him, and they were more and more happy to do for him. He didn't finish high school, and just stayed home after that.

As he was growing up, his sisters started to marry and leave the home. As his caretakers were less available, Brian was called upon to do more for himself. Despite the mother and father still helping and doing for him, he did learn to drive a car and think about getting a job. When he was in his early twenties, he was offered a job working in the stock room of a local store. While he was there, he met a girl named Amantha who was an amputee. She had apparently lost one entire leg from her hip down in a childhood accident and needed to get around on crutches. Not long after meeting, they married and set up a home. Amantha did as well as anyone could do with her handicap but still needed a lot of help. Brian, being used to being helped, rather than being the helper, quickly became overwhelmed.

Several months after the marriage, Brian came into my office accompanied by his mother and two sisters with an unusual complaint. He walked in bent over at the waist and said he could not straighten up. I examined him but could find nothing wrong. All his muscles were functioning and strong. There was no sign of atrophy, and he was well in all other respects. I ordered an MRI on his spine, and that came back completely normal. Consultation with an orthopedic surgeon revealed nothing and no diagnosis was made. I sent Brian for some physical therapy, but that did not help either. During one visit I went to a window when he left the office and watched him get into his car. He executed that just fine and straightened up as he entered.

I was beginning to think that Brian suffered from a disorder called Munchausen syndrome. This is a mental illness named for a Baron von Munchausen who was known for constantly embellishing stories about physical complaints. It is a factitious disorder where no physical reason for the symptoms are found, but the patient reveals by their attitude and behavior a strong need to convince others to believe they are really ill.

I also noted in my meetings with Brian—where he was always accompanied by his mother and several sisters and not by his wife—his unusually jovial aspect in describing his symptoms, and how eagerly his family members assisted him. Both he and the family seemed to be delighted whenever I ordered any tests that might help to elucidate the problem. When absolutely nothing turned up, I suggested that we seek consultation with a psychiatrist. As I expected, this news was not received with any enthusiasm by Brian or any of the family members.

The problem went on for months with no abatement of his symptoms. Brian quit his job and now was being supported by his amputee wife. At one visit the family came in and told me they had not followed up on my suggestion to make an appointment with a psychiatrist but instead had arranged to bring Brian to the Mayo Clinic in Cleveland where he would be in residence at the hospital and undergo an entire battery of tests. Several family members were to accompany him and stay at a nearby hotel where they could see him every day. I told them to keep me informed of their findings.

No cause for Brian's inability to straighten up was found at the Mayo Clinic either, and he was discharged without a diagnosis. Since Amantha had to work and could not adequately care for Brian, they both moved back to the family home where Brian was now cared for once again by his mother and sisters, several of whom lived nearby and came often to help. I continued to see Brian now and then, always accompanied by doting family members. One day they came in and told me that they had heard about a neurologist that had success in treating patients with similar disorders and that she was giving him weekly injections which seemed to be helping. However, the doctor told them that it was a chronic illness and that since the injections only offered temporary relief, he would have to keep receiving them. I asked what she told them was his problem, and they gave me a diagnosis with some obscure name that I had never heard of and could not find in a medical dictionary. I also asked them to tell me what injections he was receiving as since I was still his primary care physician, I needed to know this. I communicated with the neurologist by phone but when asked about the injections, I was told it was something she compounded herself. I suspect what was helping was the placebo effect of the injection. It was obvious both Brian and the family needed to believe that Brian really did have an illness and that the illness was incurable so that they could continue to take care of their baby and the baby could continue receiving the care which now he was assured he would always need. This went on as long as I remained in touch with Brian and the family, and everyone seemed happy with their roles. Brian and Amantha never had children but everyone seemed happy and content with the new set up.

The lesson for me in all this was "all's well that ends well".

Cynthia and Henry

꧁꧂

I first met Cynthia and Henry when I was called to the emergency one evening to learn that their six-year-old daughter, Candace, was suffering from a severe asthmatic attack. Since I was on call that evening for the emergency room of the hospital, all emergent calls were routed through me.

I had learned the lesson the hard way of not referring patients to specialists unless I had screened them first. One evening my husband and I were about to leave our house to attend a dinner at a friend's home to which a group of our friends were invited. Just as we were about to leave, I got a call from my answering service telling me that the mother of a patient of a doctor that I was covering had called and was very concerned that her daughter might be having an attack of appendicitis. I called the mother back, and she told me her daughter was having severe pain on the right side of her abdomen. Since it sounded like a surgical problem I was tempted to tell the mother to go to the emergency room where I would have the surgeon on call meet them.

However, at the last moment I checked myself as I knew that was not the right way to proceed and that all patients should be seen first by the primary care doctor before making a referral. Since I had a small second office in my home, I told the mother I would see them there. As they lived nearby, they arrived in a short time.

I proceeded to examine the girl, an attractive teenager who was in considerable distress. A condition which often mimics appendicitis called mittelschmerz must always be ruled out in a teenage girl. This condition sometimes occurs in the middle of the menstrual cycle by the egg bursting out of the ovary. Not everyone experiences it, but those that do report it can produce quite severe abdominal pain. It can occur either on the left or right side of the abdomen depending on which ovary was involved. I was able to rule out an acute abdomen which would present with a rigid abdomen and would signal a ruptured appendix with accompanying peritonitis. Knowing that an examination should not just be restricted to the area of complaint I listened to her lungs and was shocked at what I heard. The girl was wheezing loudly and was having a severe asthmatic attack. I then realized that her abdominal pain was caused by her incessant and violent coughing which was irritating her abdominal muscles. Upon further questioning of the mother, she acknowledged that her daughter was indeed a known asthmatic but her complaint of the severe abdominal pain had thrown her off the track.

I prescribed medication and arranged to see her the next day and breathed a sigh of relief at not having made a surgical referral without seeing the patient first. I had saved myself considerable embarrassment and might even have saved the girl from unnecessary surgery. One thing we are taught in medical school is how difficult it is to always be accurate in making the diagnosis of appendicitis. Rarely does a patient always present with the signs and symptoms described in our textbooks. We are told that suspicion is enough to suggest surgery because it is far better to do an unnecessary surgical procedure than not to do a necessary one and risk a case of a burst appendix with accompanying peritonitis.

That experience reinforced in me the determination to always adhere to the policy of seeing a patient before making a referral. Patients would often call my office asking for a referral to a specialist. Most managed care companies required a patient to get a referral from their primary care physician before they could go to a specialist. When the secretary told them they would have to be seen first by me, they got annoyed as they wanted to go directly to a specialist and didn't want to make what they viewed as an unnecessary visit.

This policy of mine paid off countless times as it frequently happened that, when I saw the patient, I discovered they were misdiagnosing themselves and going to the wrong specialist. And just as often they didn't even require the services of a specialist as it was a condition I was more than capable of treating myself.

Candace was indeed having a severe asthma attack and so was admitted to the hospital for treatment. She did well, and I was able to discharge her several days later. I continued to see the family after she was discharged.

One day I read in a local newspaper that seventeen of the policemen from a neighboring town had won the state lottery. The total amount of the prize was fifty-three-million dollars. I was thrilled to learn this as quite a few of the policemen and their families were patients of mine. Shortly before this news was received, Candace's father came into my office requesting a referral to a urologist for a vasectomy. He and his wife Cynthia had decided they didn't want any more children. So I made the referral.

About four months later, Cynthia came into the office complaining of being tired all the time and feeling very nauseous in the mornings which was sometimes accompanied by vomiting. I examined her and didn't find anything wrong. I questioned her as to whether she could be pregnant, and she said that was impossible because Henry had had a vasectomy. Nevertheless, I thought a test to rule out pregnancy should be done despite her protesting that was not necessary. I did it nevertheless, and it was positive.

I then questioned further and asked as delicately as I could whether she might have been sexually involved with another man, and she shook her head vigorously and denied it. Henry her husband was sitting out in the waiting room, and we called him in to deliver the news. He was totally shocked and seemed as displeased as Cynthia to learn this. He affirmed that he had in fact had the vasectomy but when I questioned him if he had gone for his six week checkup to confirm that it had worked, he blushed and admitted that he did not.

Everyone was quite speechless at this news, including myself, but I thought I would lighten the atmosphere by changing the subject and asking how they had reacted to the lottery bonanza. I knew he was one of the winning po-licemen as the newspaper had listed the names of the winners. He smiled and said they were delighted but it wasn't changing their lives very much. Certainly it had added a few luxuries, a new car, renovation work on their house, a savings account for their daughter's eventual college tuition, and a planned vacation, but they were both remaining at their jobs which they loved and had no plans for any major changes in their lives. Subsequent meetings with some of the other policemen winners produced a similar response.

Shortly thereafter, they left the office after I told them to contact me soon and let me know their plans. I knew they would go through with the pregnancy despite not having planned for it. When Cynthia called to tell me that, I made a referral to a local obstetrician for management of her pregnancy. Since she was older than thirty-five, her pregnancy would be considered high risk.

I didn't see them again for about six months when the hospital called to tell me that Cynthia delivered a baby girl and that they had requested me to do the infant care. I left shortly after to check the new baby who was full term and doing just fine. I didn't know what to expect, though, when I entered the mother's room to tell her that. I must admit I was pleasantly surprised to see all three family members—Henry, Cynthia and Candace—in excellent spirits and very happy. They were thrilled and delighted with the new addition to their family and in no way exhibited the distress and disappointment they exhibited when they first learned the news of Cynthia's pregnancy.

I have seen this occur in other families as well. The news of an unplanned pregnancy usually engenders shock and mixed emotions, but the arrival of the baby is almost always a happy occasion. I have even seen the disappointment in fathers who desperately wanted a son quickly turn to delight with their new daughters.

Another case of "all's well that ends well".

Stephanie

❦

The phone rang, jarring me out of a deep sleep and interrupting a dream of lying on a sun-drenched sandy shore washed by warm, crystal clear waters. As I reached for the phone, I opened one sleepy eye and glanced at the luminous dials of the clock sitting on the night table next to my bed. Eleven o'clock! I had been asleep only an hour and a half.

I had returned earlier that evening from a full day at the office. Actually, my day had begun even earlier than that with hospital rounds at 7 A.M. Then on to the office at 9 A.M. This was February, and we were right in the midst of flu season, so the day was filled with feverish, aching, sneezing, coughing people who looked to me to make them better quickly so they could return to work the next day and not lose pay. I find practicing medicine in this season the most difficult as there is little more I can do to help except to suggest they stay home and rest and wait it out. This was in the day before antiviral medications became available. At that time, about all I could offer was symptomatic relief which, with a little effort, they can find themselves lining the supermarket shelves. So the day is filled with my dispensing advice which their mothers could have told them, and dealing with disgruntled patients who, after dragging themselves out of bed and sitting in the waiting room, are now told to go back home and go back to bed and that I don't have a miracle medicine up my sleeve. Because, if I did, as I have frequently told them, I would not be sitting in my humble office worrying about meeting my overhead, managing the paperwork for the HMOs, and whether I will catch the illness myself, but I would be on my way to Sweden to receive the Nobel Prize for Medicine.

With only a brief break for lunch, which I ate at my desk while reading lab reports, the office hours lasted until 8 P.M. I still had some calls to return and did not actually leave until 8:30 P.M. I was hungry when I got home but too tired to do anything more than grab a slice of leftover cold pizza and wolf it down before my eyelids began to droop.

I surrendered to sleep knowing that I was on call for three other practices that night and I'd better grab some ZZZZZZZs while I could.

As expected, the call was from the Emergency Room of our local hospital. I was put through after holding for about ten minutes or so while wondering, if they called me, why was I the one doing the waiting? I had nearly fallen asleep again, while holding the phone, and was jarred awake a second time by the loud voice of the ER physician on duty. He had just come on for the 11 P.M. to 7 A.M. shift so he was wide awake. He began by apologizing to me for keeping me on hold, but he said the ER was like a zoo that night and he had to receive report from the physician that was going off duty.

After a brief summary of the case, it was apparent that I had to go in to see the patient. He described a situation which sounded like it could be an acute abdomen in a teenage girl. He told me the patient's name, but it was unfamiliar to me. Most likely this was the patient of one of the doctors I was covering that night. For a brief moment I considered turning this over to the surgeon on call as the most likely cause of the problem would be appendicitis with or without rupture. In any event, the surgeon would handle it, and I could go back to my very pleasant beach dream. However, reason and responsibility prevailed, as we had been taught in our training that the differential diagnosis of abdominal pain is lengthy and there was no substitute for a good history and thorough physical. I also recalled another time in the distant past when I was similarly tempted in another case of abdominal pain which also, over the phone, sounded like a classic case of appendicitis. However, when that child was checked, it turned out to be an asthmatic attack, and the abdominal pain was caused by the irritation of the musculature of the abdominal wall from incessant coughing. In giving the history over the phone the mother never mentioned the coughing, as the young girl was a chronic asthmatic and coughed nearly all the time. However, when the child complained of abdominal pain, this being a new symptom, the mother got concerned and called. In that case, calling the surgeon might have resulted in unnecessary surgery, or at the least, a wasted visit and considerable embarrassment for me for missing the diagnosis. Of course, had the patient been known to me, I would no doubt have questioned about her asthmatic state.

That was a lesson not easily forgotten, and I remembered it as I told the ER doctor to arrange for some blood and urine studies and an abdominal X-ray and that I would be in shortly.

It didn't take me long to get ready as I had fallen asleep in my clothing, a habit picked up from internship and residency days when we slept in the on-call rooms of the hospital and had to be ready to act on a moment's notice. Also, with the limited number of on-call rooms, very often we shared the room with a member of the opposite sex so remaining in our clothes tended to avoid distractions from our duties.

I kissed my sleeping husband on the forehead and told him I was on my way to the ER. He murmured a response which I'm sure he would have no recollection of in the morning. I then headed out into the night. A light snow was falling, and by now I'm wide awake enough to enjoy the peaceful wintry scene. However, that peace is soon shattered when I remember that before the snow there was icy rain and the snow has just been covering up some very dangerous road conditions. This is confirmed to me when I arrive at the ER and notice several local ambulances and police cars parked outside. I also notice a shiny new Rolls-Bentley parked in the lot which stands out like a sore thumb among the assorted wrecks, rent-a-cars, and compacts which surround it. Our community hospital serves a large, very economically diverse community. The catchment area contains everything from low income housing, the so-called Mt. Laurel housing, to the homes surrounding some of the lakes and golf courses in the area which sell for up to several million dollars. I took a moment to admire the Rolls, then quickly murmured my usual prayer for God's guidance before I left my car to enter the ER.

The ER physician was correct. The ER was indeed like a zoo. The CB radio was blasting with messages from ambulances on their way in with accident victims. The ER doc ignored me as I entered, as he was occupied barking instructions over the two-way radios to the rescue workers riding the ambulances. I tried to attract his attention, but he just waved me away, pointing to the back of the ER, I still didn't know to what. Not a nurse was to be seen; all were, I'm sure, occupied in the individual cubicles, which I could tell by the name plates on the doors were all filled. I weaved my way past the portable X-ray machines, heart monitors, crash carts with defibrillators, patients lying on stretchers, and crying, stunned relatives, to the desk where, on a wall, many clipboards hung from a corkboard. I had already forgotten the last name of the patient I am there to see, but fortunately I do remember her first name, Stephanie. I located a clipboard with the name Stephanie Ann Warner next to the name of the Dr. I am covering for that evening. The chief complaint is listed as "abdominal pain", so this must be the patient. But there is no room number on the chart. Where is the patient, then?

I enter one of the cubicles to find a nurse who is attending to someone on a respirator. She tells me she has been with this patient for the last two hours and cannot help me. I enter another cubicle where the nurse is attending to a comatose patient with an N-G tube in place. The other end of the tube is attached to a large syringe sitting in a basin of ice water. An overdose, no doubt, as they are performing a gastric lavage to extract the swallowed substance. This nurse cannot help me either.

Finally, I noticed someone sitting alone on a bench huddled up into a ball, her face hidden in her lap. I approached and asked her if she is Stephanie Warner. She slowly looked up, and I saw a very pretty, tear-streaked face which obviously, not too long before, had been made up to the nines.

Her mascara and eyeliner, though smeared, had been carefully applied and her lipstick was accented by lip liner. This was a girl who spent a lot of time in front of the mirror. Her clothing was rumpled but stylish and expensive, and her handbag had little G's all over, no doubt a Gucci. The pinched, flushed look of her face and the dullness of her eyes told me she was in a lot of pain, and probably feverish. I glanced down again at the clipboard and reviewed the brief history and vital signs noted by the admitting nurse. Her temperature was indeed elevated at 103 degrees Fahrenheit, but this time I noted the patient's age. I am stunned to see that she is only twelve. For a moment I wonder why she is alone and how she got here, but my first priority is to find out what is going on. Once again, I looked around for a nurse to assist the patient to a room or at least a stretcher, so I can examine her. As there is still no one in sight who is available to help, I offer to get her a wheelchair and then took her to a room down the hall which is reserved for psychiatric emergencies, but was then free. She firmly declines the wheelchair and begins to walk, doubled over, toward the room which I have indicated. Somehow, with great difficulty, she gets there and gingerly sets herself down again on the low stretcher. The care with which she lowers herself on to the stretcher is a bad sign to me, as it signals peritoneal irritation and a possible abdominal or pelvic emergency. The list of possibilities runs through my mind: ruptured appendix, ruptured ovarian

cyst, peritonitis, toxic megacolon, severe infection of the gynecologic system and impending abortion—in any event all very
serious. I also consider a ruptured ectopic pregnancy, but put
this lower down on my list because of the patient's age.

There is a light rap on the door and the ward clerk enters
with the lab results. I quickly review them and note that her
white count is 31,000, a roughly fivefold increase from what
is normal. I question the clerk about who brought the patient.
The clerk says she was signed in by her mother but she
doesn't know where she is now, but is sure she is "around". I
firmly instruct her to find her without delay, as I probably
will need to do a pelvic exam and I prefer to do it with the
mother's presence and consent. I also wonder if the girl can
give me a reliable history considering her age. I questioned
her nevertheless. How long have you been ill? Answer:
Missed school for past three days. I question further about
vomiting, diarrhea, vaginal discharge. She nods only to vaginal discharge so now I know I need to know more about her
sexual history. It was somewhat uncomfortable for me to ask
this of a twelve-year-old, but her openness and willingness
to answer all my questions surprised me. Usually I am either
lied to or, at best, get evasive answers. Stephanie told me
that she has been sexually active since age ten, has had many
sexual partners, and volunteered that she "hangs out a lot
on the west side of New York". I try to hide my shock at
hearing her story especially as, having trained in a ghetto

hospital, her story was not all that unusual. However, in our suburban community, far away from the ghetto, it was unusual. It was not necessary to pose too many questions to Stephanie as, despite her pain, she was quite happy to tell all the lurid details of her "past". I learn that her last period was two weeks before, so I mentally put a light scratch through the ectopic pregnancy diagnosis, which is now a lot less likely. As she is telling me that has been treated several times for gonorrhea and several other venereal diseases, the door opened and in walked a beautiful, well-groomed woman bearing a striking resemblance to Stephanie. I realize this must be her mother. I smile a greeting and she gives me a polite, disinterested smile back. I ask her what has been happening with Stephanie, but Stephanie quickly interrupts to say that she doesn't know anything as she has been "out of town" for the past few days and has just gotten home. Stephanie apparently has been with her housekeeper who didn't know anything was wrong.

Laughingly, Stephanie says that the housekeeper, who is supposed to also be her babysitter, always goes off to the room right after dinner and therefore doesn't know that Stephanie leaves the house soon after. This occurs several nights a week. Sometimes she is picked up by another girlfriend who is old enough to drive, or a boyfriend, or if they are not available, she takes the bus into New York City. And, since the housekeeper has a hearing problem, she doesn't know when

Stephanie leaves or returns to the house early in the morning. Then, after just a few hours' sleep, Stephanie goes to school. Her teachers on several occasions have reported her for falling asleep in class, but no follow up was made as somehow Stephanie has managed to avoid getting failing grades.

I watched Stephanie's mother as she was relating this story, but her face remained impassive. It occurred to me that she might be on drugs, as she seemed totally indifferent to what Stephanie was relating.

With the mother's consent, I then proceeded with my physical examination which revealed extreme tenderness throughout her abdomen, which was especially tender in her pelvic area. Fortunately she did not exhibit abdominal rigidity which would have alerted me to peritonitis, a medical emergency with a high fatality rate. I declined to perform an internal examination but did obtain a specimen of vaginal discharge which was sent to the lab for analysis.

Stephanie was admitted to the hospital with a presumptive diagnosis of pelvic inflammatory disease and placed on high doses of two antibiotics administered intravenously. Since it would take two days to get the culture results back from the lab, the antibiotics chosen were broad spectrum and which most often worked well in this clinical setting.

As I was telling Stephanie's mother my plan to admit her daughter to the hospital for treatment, the man accompanying Stephanie's mother appeared. The disinterest he exhibited in everything that was going on led me to believe he was not Stephanie's father. He whispered in the mother's ear and tugged gently at her sleeve, and they both left soon after. Before departing, Stephanie's mother gave her a quick kiss on her forehead and said she would be in to visit her when she had a free moment.

Stephanie told her regular doctor she wanted me to continue her care while in the hospital, so I remained with the case. During her stay in the hospital, Stephanie underwent an MRI which confirmed the diagnosis. The study revealed that her fallopian tubes were filled with fluid and there was also free fluid within the pelvic cavity. Her cultures revealed a mixed infection with Chlamydia and Gonorrhea.

Since it appeared to me that this young girl was the victim of extreme neglect despite growing up in a financially secure household, I reported the case to the division of Youth and Family Services. They came promptly to see Stephanie in the hospital and called in the mother to their office as well. When questioned about the father, they were told he left them many years before. The person who interviewed the mother made a note about her flat affect and uncooperativeness and so made a strong recommendation that the mother undergo treatment as they were certain she was using drugs. After several interviews with both Stephanie and her mother, it was decided that Stephanie be placed in foster care. The arrangement was to be temporary, pending the mother's participation in the recommended treatment regimen.

After fourteen days on IV therapy, another MRI was performed which showed resolution of the problem. She celebrated her thirteenth birthday during her hospital stay, and I arranged for a cake for her to share with the nursing staff. I called her mother to tell her of the impending celebration, but she was not available and didn't call me back. I left the message with the housekeeper. Everyone sang "Happy Birthday," but her mother never showed up to join us. In fact, she had visited Stephanie only once during the entire fourteen days and only for a few minutes even then.

Stephanie was discharged to the home of the foster parents who came to pick her up. When I met with them, I felt comfortable about discharging her to their care as I felt they were both caring and responsible people. They also had an impeccable record of administering prior foster care and had excellent ratings. Stephanie was happy to be leaving the hospital and reacted very positively to her meeting with the foster parents. She was all smiles upon discharge, and the staff gave her a rousing send off.

At this point Stephanie was lost to my care, but not to my thoughts as I could not help thinking with great sadness of the likeliness that Stephanie would be infertile, as the inevitable scarring of her fallopian tubes would not allow for successful fertilization and implantation of a fertilized egg. How terribly sad that, at the age of twelve—or nearly thirteen as she kept reminding me—such a prediction was almost a certainty.

Henrietta and Murray

❧ⓖ☙

Henrietta had been my patient for at least a decade before she finally felt comfortable and secure enough in my presence to talk openly and freely to me. I had long noted her sad appearance and attempted to question her about her life when she came in for minor ailments, but she always answered in monosyllables and never revealed anything beyond the sore throat or minor bellyache which brought her in.

I always felt it was important to know something about the lives of my patients so that I could be more effective in rendering their medical care. So, upon the first meeting with a patient and taking their medical history, as well as learning about any illnesses or surgeries they had, it was also important to know their family history. Employment history was also important to know as they might be exposed to dangerous substances. However, a question I always asked at the end of taking their medical history always elicited a wide eyed, shocked response. That question was: "And what do you do for fun?" After their shock wore off, they often were delighted to tell me something about their hobbies and avocations. As for me, I felt I really got to know the person and it developed a bond with them which was important in their treatment. Upon subsequent visits I would ask them about their hobbies and pastimes and they enjoyed telling me.

However, on this one day that I once again tried to engage Henrietta in a conversation, she broke down sobbing and started to tell me what was going on in her life. She had been married for about fifteen years and regretfully never had had any children. She was a full time homemaker and had never worked during her marriage. She then described to me a usual evening spent with her husband.

She said he frequently came home late and at unexpected times even though she knew he clocked out from the factory where he worked the same time every night. On those nights he would park the car on their grass, and come into the house reeking of alcohol. She would serve him his dinner which she had kept warm for him in the oven, and he would open another bottle of wine which he often brought home with him, as he knew she would not serve him any. He would barely eat the dinner but would drink copious amounts of the wine. Shortly after dinner, he would begin to attack and criticize her, and criticize the appearance of their home. Often he would begin to throw and break things. Then he would vomit all over himself and pass out on the floor.

After he passed out, Henrietta told me she would spend the rest of the evening cleaning up the house, removing his soiled clothing and replacing them with clean pajamas. All this done, she would somehow get him into the bed, and then go out on the lawn and park his car in the street so that the neighbors would not see the car on the lawn the next morning and know the condition in which he came home the night before. I never met the husband, but she described him as being a large man, which made it unbelievable to me that this frail little lady could manage to get her husband off the floor and into the bed. But she said she did it, and I believed her. Apparently this went on several times a week for a number of years.

I suggested she get help and attend Al-Alon meetings in our area and gave her a list of locations where they met. She took the list, but I did not get the feeling that she would follow up.

I did not see her for another year. This time she did not require prompting to talk about her situation. She told me that nothing had changed and that the same scenario that she previously described was still occurring and perhaps now with even more frequency. She also mentioned that his job might be in danger as he had been called on the carpet several times for poor performance and even once for falling asleep at the machine that he worked. She kept saying over and over again, "What am I doing wrong, what am I doing wrong?" I repeated to her the Al-Anon mantra of the three C's. You didn't cause it, you can't change it, and you can't cure it. And once again, I made a strong recommendation to attend the Al-Anon meetings and assured her that she would get the kind of help she needed there. I also suggested that after attending a few meetings she come in and tell me what she thought of the help that was offered.

A few weeks later she came into the office again and told me she had been to several meetings. I asked her if they made any suggestions that might be helpful. She told me that they suggested that she stop cleaning up after him and that the only hope she had for anything changing would be to allow him to experience the consequences of the havoc he was creating. I repeated that several times to her: Consequences are the only things that have any chance of bringing about any change. So long as she keeps cleaning up after him, that is, removing the consequences, he has no reason to change and she is enabling him to continue his behavior. I could see in the brightening of her facial expression that this line of reasoning was beginning to make inroads. However, I did not yet feel confident that she had the strength to follow this advice. So I told her to keep attending the meetings and even to seek a sponsor there.

Several months later she came into the office once again but this time smiling and looking considerably more attractive as it was the first time I had seen her with a pretty dress and wearing makeup. I asked her what was going on, and she told me that with the Al-Anon help and support from her sponsor she was able to finally follow their suggestion to stop cleaning up after him. So one night when he once again came home drunk after parking the car on their lawn, she served him a cold supper and then after he once again vomited and passed out on the floor, she left him there. So when he woke up the next morning on the floor, in his clothes covered with vomit and then saw his car parked on the lawn, he was speechless and went to clean himself up. When he left the house to go to work, he noticed several neighbors looking over his way and smiling which seemed to be a great embarrassment to him.

This same scenario went on for several more nights where she said she did not clean up after him, and finally he came to her and admitted he needed treatment. The Al-Anon people had already given her the names of several treatment centers in their area, and she passed this to him and told him to make the arrangements.

Her husband entered a thirty-day inpatient treatment program, and she told me he had just gotten his three months sober pin from the Alcoholics Anonymous group he attends. Henrietta keeps going to the Al-Anon meetings which she says she now enjoys. She is even looking forward to being someone's sponsor one day. She thanked me profusely for turning her in the direction which in turn has helped her to turn her life in a better direction. I was pleased to see this now attractive, smiling lady leave my office that day.

Henrietta's story reminded me of something similar that I had experienced when I was a new mother, before I had attended medical school and before I knew anything about enabling. My son Murray, around the age of one year or so, had developed the ability to make himself vomit. After his dinner I would put him into his crib where he would stand and jump up and down obviously not wanting me to leave the room so he could go to sleep. Shortly after I put him in the crib, he would proceed to vomit all over his clean sleep suit, the sheets in the crib, and the floor. My husband I and would then start to clean him up, change his sleep clothes, change the sheets on the bed and then mop up the floor, and all the while my son was jumping up and down gleefully in the crib, happy that all this activity bought him another forty-five minutes of the "fun" of staying awake. This went on night after night. My husband and I were getting frantic. We didn't know how to stop it. One night we were so exhausted we decided to just leave him in the mess. I suppose when he saw we were not coming in to do the usual clean up, he lay down and soon fell asleep. This went on for a few more nights. I would put him clean and fresh into his crib after dinner, and shortly thereafter he would again vomit and mess up everything around him. But, once again we did not go into his room to clean up and left him in the mess. And would you believe it, after about three or four more nights he stopped vomiting. Apparently by coming into the room and doing the cleanup which bought him another forty-five minutes of "fun," we were enabling him to continue the behavior. When we left him with the consequences, the mess, he stopped doing it. I know some parents would consider this unspeakably cruel behavior but I suppose that is what is called "tough love", and it worked even with a one-year-old child.

Many times, in the course of addiction treatment it is necessary to suggest the employment of "tough love" techniques. Most of the significant others find this very difficult to do as it goes against what our loving instincts dictate to us to do. But we have to make them realize that the only hope they have for change is to allow the addict to feel the consequences. Yes, at times the consequences are very severe, leading to loss of a job, the breakup of a marriage, jail time, and even death. But so long as someone is made comfortable in a behavior they have no reason to go through the pain of change. The idea is to make them uncomfortable by allowing them to fully experience the consequences.

Freddie and Courtney

✌◈◈✍

I have grouped these two stories together because they both illustrate the same problem not infrequently encountered in a medical setting.

There are times when an unpleasant diagnosis must be given to a patient or caretaker. When this was necessary, I always tried to give it with honesty but also with sensitivity, compassion, and most importantly, hope. I always felt it was important to hold out hope even with the most dire of diagnoses. We have all heard stories of patients who were told they had three months to live and lived another thirty years. That is not to say that it is not necessary to be honest and stay in reality, but it is possible at the same time to present a plan and alternatives that are not hopeless.

The receipt of such an unpleasant diagnosis engenders many different reactions in people. Some give up no matter what you say, some summon up all their courage from the depths and tell you they are willing to do anything no matter how remote the outcome, and some, not liking the message, want to kill the messenger.

It was the latter reaction I encountered with these two patients, but in these two cases, the reaction was not in the patient but rather in their caretakers.

Freddie was a little boy, brought in by his mother one day asking me to perform a physical examination which was required by the pre-school program in which she planned to enroll him. His regular physician had not been available to, so she asked me to do it. As soon as I met with them in the examination room, I immediately had the feeling that something was amiss here, as when the mother told me he was four years old, I had a sense that he didn't look at all like all the other four-year-olds I cared for. A regular part of a physical examination of a child is to get their height and weight and then that would be plotted on a growth chart to see how they compare with other children the same age. Since this could differ from one culture to another, we used different charts for Caucasian and Asian children. Freddie was way off the chart for a four-year-old male. His height and weight were more in line with measurements we would expect of a two-year-old. I completed the examination and then sat down with the mother and told her of my findings: that Freddie did not seem to be growing properly and some studies to find out why would be appropriate. She sat in stunned silence and made no response to what I was saying. Since I seemed to make no inroads with her, I resolved to send my findings to his regular physician for follow up. The mother and child left the office immediately after, and the mother made no further comments to me.

About a half hour later, I became aware there was a big commotion going on in the waiting room. Apparently the father of the child had stormed in and was shouting and insisting on seeing me and berating me for telling the mother what I said about his son not growing properly. I tried to talk him down but got no place with that and since he was getting more and more belligerent and even violent, I signaled to the secretary to call the police, which she had already started to do even before I signaled. They arrived within minutes and ushered the father out of the office. Several days later I informed their regular physician of my findings, but when he contacted the parents he encountered a similar reaction. So he told me that he had to refer the case to the Division of Youth and Family Services for follow up. At that point, both their physician and I lost contact with the family. I can only hope that Freddie was referred for proper follow up care and that the cause of his failure to thrive was elucidated and treated.

Courtney also came to me because her regular physician was not available. According to her mother, she needed a physical to participate in sports in the high school she attended.

When I met with them in the examination room, I noticed that Courtney had very poor color and seemed very lethargic for a teenager. She also seemed disinterested in the conversation that her mother and I had as I took her history, and she picked at her fingernails continually. I also noticed that although it was a warm day outside, she seemed to have several layers of clothing on which just drooped on her body. The mother told me that she was also under the care of a gynecologist and a gastroenterologist as well as their primary care physician. I questioned about each of the specialists, and her mother told me that she was seeing the gynecologist because of her arrested menses and the gastroenterologist because of stomach pains. When I asked further about their findings, I was told "they were still doing tests".

I asked the mother if she would wait in the waiting room while I did my physical examination, and she left the room to sit there. It is my practice to see teenagers without the parent in the room because I need to ask health-related questions which they might be reluctant to answer truthfully if the parent was present. However, if I find it necessary to perform an internal exam, I would then require the presence of the mother.

I gave Courtney a gown and asked her to remove all her clothing while I left the room. When I came back in, she had not done this. When I asked why, she said none of her other doctors asked her to do this. I told her I could not perform a proper physical and would not be able to sign her form until she did this. So she started to remove her clothing but placed them on the examination table next to her. When I lifted the clothing to put them on the chair, I noticed that they were unusually heavy.

I started the exam with her height and weight and saw that her height was five feet, six inches but that she only weighed eighty pounds. Her height rate was very slow, and her skin was unusually dry and flaky.

I felt that this was an emergency situation as this girl was in great danger from her obvious anorexia, so I called the mother in and told her that I advised immediate hospitalization in the eating disorders unit of our hospital. The mother became irate at hearing this news and told me that she was already under the care of other doctors and that all she asked me for was a physical and to sign her form. Without further discussion they quickly departed from the office. I placed an immediate call to the director of the eating disorders unit for advice as to how to effectively proceed with this case as I felt the girl was in imminent danger. He suggested I report the case immediately to the Division of Youth and Family Services which I did.

I heard no follow up about the girl, but several weeks later I got a letter from the New Jersey Medical Society. Apparently the mother had reported me for inconsiderate, alarming, and reckless behavior in the care I rendered to her daughter. Fortunately I had documented good notes about my findings along with my prompt reporting to the eating disorders unit and DYFS which cleared me of any malpractice accusations, and the Medical Society immediately dropped the case. In further thinking about the case, I realized the girl's clothing felt unusually heavy because heavy things were in her pockets. She must have done this hoping I would not ask her to undress and then would not notice her extreme weight loss. Anorectic patients often resort to similar schemes to disguise their extreme weight loss.

Another instance of "if you hate the message, kill the messenger".

Adrianne and Bill

೦ഗ৩৩৩

Adrianne had recently had her fourth child in six years. She was married to Bill who was a real estate agent in our town and had in fact done the transaction which enabled me to purchase the building in which my office was housed. So, I knew Bill quite well but had only recently become acquainted with Adrianne and their children. Bill was a very successful agent, very capable and especially charming. I even felt at times during our transactions that he was somewhat flirtatious. His family had previously been patients of the doctor whose building and practice I had purchased, and they had decided to continue their care with me.

One day Adrianne came into the office with the newest baby who was then about six months old. She came in tow with the other three, a two-year-old girl whom she balanced in her other arm and two other children, three- and four-year-old boys whom she brought into the office in a double stroller. Apparently they had been driven to the office by taxi, with which they had also arranged to pick them up after they had concluded their visit in the office.

The nurse brought Adrianne and the six-month-old into our baby room for his well baby care and immunizations. As our baby room was very small, the staff cared for and tried to amuse the three others because they could not all fit in the room and an exam would not have been possible with the distraction the other children would have made. The visit with the newborn was routine. The baby was still being nursed and was thriving well. I couldn't help noticing that Adrianne, who was actually a very pretty woman, had gained weight and looked very disheveled. She was wearing a sweat shirt and pants and no makeup, and looked very exhausted. I commented that it must be very difficult caring for four young children, all too young to attend school, and home with her all the time. I questioned her about whether she had any help—family members or Bill himself—and pointed out that a nursing mother needed a lot of rest. In the old days, when extended families lived together, all the nursing mother had to do was nurse and care for the infant while family members helped with everything else, including the care of the other children.

But these were different times. Families were often scattered and unavailable to new mothers and this was so in Adrianne and Bill's case.

Adrianne responded to my questioning by saying that there were no family members nearby and that Bill was working very hard and often did not get home from his office until two o'clock in the morning. He said this was because he was unable to work at home because of all the noise the children made. A mini alarm went off in my head when she told me this, as I thought it quite unusual for a realtor to be working those hours as he certainly was not meeting with clients or showing properties then. Also, saying he had to work so late in his office because of all the noise the children made was difficult to believe as they were all in bed and asleep by 7 P.M.

I questioned Adrianne as to why she did not hire someone to help her. I pointed out that Bill had an acknowledged reputation as a successful realtor in the area and must be doing very well judging by the long hours he was working. Her eyes opened wide as I said this, and she nodded her head in agreement and said, yes, he was doing very well. But, she said, she didn't think the children would accept being cared for by a stranger. I suggested that she question neighbors about hiring someone or advertise to get someone, and conduct interviews and check references. Once having selected someone, she could bring them in to get them acquainted with the children and the household while she was still there so the children could adjust to the presence of the newcomer and Adrianne could see how they reacted. And then, in small doses, leave them with the new housekeeper for gradually extended periods. I then suggested she could use the free time to do things for herself. I pointed out that a person needed to fill themselves up before they had anything to give away.

Adrianne reacted to my suggestions with a big smile, as if it were something she had already wished for, but now was being given permission to do. She said she would talk to Bill about this and even said that with all the people he knew perhaps he could help her find someone.

I didn't see Adrianne again for several months, until once again she brought in the youngest infant for his well baby care and immunizations. However, I noticed this time that Adrianne had not arrived with the other three children. When I questioned her about them, she said that they were at a day care center which had recently just opened and were soon to be picked up by her new housekeeper. I also noticed that Adrianne had lost weight, was no longer nursing, and looked absolutely lovely. She was well groomed, wearing a fashionable blouse and slacks, and had on makeup and a beautifully arranged hairdo. She looked very pretty, was spirited, and didn't look at all fatigued.

I questioned her some about her family life, wondering whether Bill was still working those late hours, and she said, no, he wasn't and was coming home each night earlier and having dinner with the family. She seemed so much happier and thanked me profusely for suggesting that she get help.

Once again, by paying attention to the family dynamic and not limiting myself only to the patient at hand—in this case, the infant—I was able to intervene and hopefully prevent what sounded like and I feared was a potentially dangerous situation. I never knew or found out why Bill was working those very suspect late hours, but I suppose "all's well that ends well". I suspected that Adrianne actually really wanted to do what I suggested, but needed the permission or "okay" from someone in presumed authority to give it to her.

Victor and Daphne

❧

During the many years that I practiced medicine I was often consulted by patients to help with problems in their lives beyond treating their sore throats and bellyaches. So, there were many occasions wherein quite a number of people confessed and sought help with a variety of problems in their lives. These ranged from marital problems where a wife learned her husband was having an affair, with problems dealing with homosexual urges in people involved in heterosexual relationships and even marriages, with discovering crossdressing in loved ones and children, and many other intimate details that no one else was privy to.

There are many people who wouldn't go to a psychiatrist or psychologist if you offered it to them for free, as they believed there was some sort of stigma attached to it, i.e., they must be crazy. But they would talk to their priest or their doctor. I had enough trouble getting them to go to a specialist in the rare events when I needed to send them. When I suggested consulting with a specialist on a particular problem they would often say, "Oh, can't you take care of it, Doc?" They were so trusting, I believe they would have let me do brain surgery in the office.

And so, knowing that about my patients, I would agree to at least listen and help where I felt I could. The two stories that I will describe in this chapter were among the most difficult to deal with as their novelty created in me a feeling of insecurity in dealing with them. I had never tackled problems like this before. However, as the people said they trusted me and really had no other way of dealing with the problem, I said that I would listen and give it a try.

The first was a young Chinese man who had not long before imported a wife from China. She didn't speak a word of English, and the husband was not much better. He explained to me that neither of them knew anything about sex as it was a forbidden subject when they were growing up. They wanted a family but didn't know how to proceed. So I dug out from a closet some models of female genital anatomy and tried to explain. I also saw the wife alone and by gesture and pictures and by encouraging her own self-exploration, I tried to explain further. The wife smiled and even laughed throughout all this, which I realized was the manifestation of her shyness. I encouraged her to continue this self-exploration and not be afraid as she would not hurt herself. Then I met with the husband. Helping him to get familiar with his body and what it could do was somewhat more difficult as he was even more shy than the wife. But with patience and gentleness, and always being totally professional so that it could feel this was purely clinical and not necessarily a prohibited activity, he began to relax somewhat with it all. I taught him self-stimulation to create an erection which I explained was necessary for penetration.

We made another appointment for two weeks, and they arrived promptly. I asked how they were proceeding, and they described moderate success with their separate endeavors but had not yet tried anything together. I urged them to continue what they were doing, but added an activity of exploring each other without yet attempting penetration. I suggested they do this for another month and to do it at least several times a week. I also suggested it be done under the covers but without any clothing on and with touching each other to a point of toleration. As soon as one became uncomfortable, they were told to stop.

A month later I saw them both again. But this time, I not only saw them together but I also met with them individually. Again with a few words but mainly gestures the wife nodded enthusiastically in response. She seemed less shy and more comfortable in my presence and made more eye

contact. Her smiles now seemed more to be of acknowl-
edgement and gratitude than purely of shyness. I told them
to continue what they were doing, but now she was to add
self-penetration with her fingers. As for the husband, he
too seemed to be less shy, and he smiled broadly when I
complimented them on their progress. The new activity I
suggested to him was to self-stimulate beyond mere erection but to achieve orgasm. However, when I suggested this
he conveyed to me that he had already done that. So instead I added the new activity of trying to penetrate his wife
with his fingers. He nodded enthusiastically and continued
to smile broadly. Some part of me started to think he was
really beginning to enjoy this and not see it purely as a
duty. Another appointment for one month was made.

Once again, they arrived at the duly appointed time.
The wife was acquiring a few more words in English and
seemed to better understand me. She seemed to excel in
saying "thank you" and responded with it to most everything I said. They had successfully accomplished everything I had suggested in the last visit, and so I thought it
might be time to make an approach to the full monty. I described the position I wanted them to assume, while cau-
tioning the husband not to put his full weight on his wife.
After he achieved erection he was to attempt penetration
but only to an inch or so within her. He could make several
attempts but no more. Each time they tried this, he could

try to penetrate somewhat more. I prepared the wife by suggesting the use of a lubricant but also made her realize that at first this might be somewhat painful and blood might appear, but not to worry. I also encouraged the wife to help him achieve erection by touching him and encouraged him to continue to use finger penetration of his wife. Once again we made an appointment for another month.

A month later they came in, holding hands and smiling, and reported they had been successful in full penetration. By their broad smiles showing all their teeth, I realized that the activity was no longer seen as a duty but by now seemed to be a source of enjoyment for them. I told them to continue what they were doing and even placed a gold star on them, which I kept for children after vaccinations. That made them smile even more broadly, which I didn't think was possible.

A year later they called to tell me the wife was pregnant. They didn't come into the office to tell me this because the company the husband worked for had transferred him to another city. And once again they thanked me profusely.

The second was a patient who worked for a company where I was the staff physician and so I had done his yearly physicals for the past eight years. Although I only saw him once a year, we had a friendly, outgoing relationship. The appointment this time, however, was not for his yearly physical, but rather for another problem that he was having.

When I questioned him further, he said that actually it was not his problem he was seeing me for, but his wife's problem. They had been married for two years, and he was very distressed because he said his wife was frigid and was always repelling his advances. He was a young, handsome virile man, and although he said he loved his wife, he found this very distressing. He then asked me if I would see her and see if I could determine the cause of the problem and hopefully treat it. I said I would see her and try to determine the root of the problem and hopefully the cure.

He made an appointment for the following week, and his wife showed up. When I met her in the examination room, I saw that she was a very beautiful woman and was impeccably dressed and made up. I asked her if she knew why her husband had made this appointment and she replied that yes, she did, and that it was because she never wanted to have sex with him.

Before launching into the problem, I questioned her about her medical and family history and then asked if she had had any sexual experiences before marriage. At first, she clammed up about this and even turned her head away. But then when she looked my way again, I could see there were tears in her eyes. I assured her that anything she told me would just remain between the two of us and was totally confidential.

She then related a story to me about her mother who divorced her father when she was very young and then took up with a boyfriend who lived with them. She was only about seven years old at the time. She said that when her mother left early in the morning to go to work he often would climb into bed with her as he did not leave for work until several hours later. She said he would put his arms around her and then put his hands all over her. There were times when he actually tried to have sex with her. She said she was frightened and wanted to scream, but he threatened to tell her mother what a bad girl she was. She developed the belief that it was her fault that this was happening and that she really was a bad girl. For that reason she never told her mother what was happening. The mother's relationship with the guy lasted for several more years, and he kept coming to her bed and became even more aggressive toward her. When she was about ten years old he forced her to have sex with him on several occasions, and she said that was extremely painful and left lasting scars on her memory.

Fortunately, the relationship between her mother and her boyfriend broke up soon after that. However, she was left with a memory of sex as a horribly painful and degrading activity, and that is why she was rejecting her husband's advances.

Her memories were so tragic and searing that I knew it would take quite a while and a lot of patience to erase these memories and make her feel secure in her husband's advances. I tried to explain that although she had had a very unfortunate experience in childhood, that things for her need not be the same again. I impressed upon her that her husband had brought her to me to help her, and that was because he loved her so much. So I instructed her to just be open and observant to his loving gestures and recognize his kindness and concern for her happiness.

I met once again with the husband, and being sworn to secrecy about what had happened to her in childhood, I just told him that she was amenable to working on the problem and that I was hopeful of our progress. But I also cautioned him it would not occur overnight and to be patient. I also suggested he refrain for the time being making any sexual advances or demands on her, but just to demonstrate in every other way his love and concern for her. He agreed to this and we made an appointment to meet again in several weeks.

At that time, I felt my attention needed to be mainly devoted to the wife, and so I only met with her. She seemed more relaxed in my presence and said she was also feeling more comfortable with her husband as he was just being loving and kind and not making sexual demands on her. At this meeting I told her that sex could be a pleasurable experience and not just the horror of what it was earlier in her life. I encouraged and instructed her to self-stimulate and then come back in and tell me how that was. Several weeks later she reported it had been scary and frightening at first but she was "okay" with it now. I also encouraged her to participate in hugging and kissing with her husband but also instructed her husband to not pressure her further than that. In time that too because pleasurable for both.

As time went on, I encouraged more pleasurable sexual activities and then to provide them for each other. Daphne was obviously starting to relax and feel more secure about all this. And apparently one night, despite my instructions, they went all the way. Daphne came into the office a few days later all smiles and said she felt a lot better about sex. Her husband was loving and very gentle, and she was able to experience pleasure and not just horror. For a while we still dealt with two steps forward and one step backward, but in time even that went away and I didn't need to see Daphne any longer. Once again I started to see the husband only for his yearly physical exams and was delighted when he gave me a thumbs up every time.

They are now the parents of four children. So I guess I can chalk that one up to a success story.

When I first consented to help these patients with their problems, I feared there might be a downside to it. However, as I knew they were uncomfortable about seeking another way of dealing with them, I agreed to try to help. I was happy to realize that in the end there was no downside to either of these cases. I felt a great deal of joy to be trusted with the intimate details of their lives and to be able to be of help to them. The long-standing relationship that you have and your approach to problems in a larger context involving other family members makes for an enhanced perspective in treatment. To me that is the uniqueness and beauty of being a Family Physician.

Darlene

⌈⌈⌈⌈⌈

Darlene was seven months old when I first saw her in my office. Apparently she had been cared for by another pediatrician since birth. Since my practice was dedicated to Family Care I was not thought of as a pediatrician, despite extensive training in that area as part of a Family Practice residency, and so I was not often recommended by the obstetricians who delivered the babies for their ongoing care. However, I often would see them later on, as was this case with Darlene.

I was the physician for the grandparents of the child when all these problems developed, and the grandparents suggested to the parents that they seek a second opinion before consenting to anything as drastic as surgery. Having often seen infants and children in my waiting room, they knew that I cared for infants and children as well as adults and even seniors.

Darlene had experienced three urinary tract infections since birth, and the pediatrician had suggested to the frantic parents that it was time to give serious consideration to corrective surgery as the frequent infections could lead to permanent damage to her kidneys. The corrective surgery being considered involved relocation of the ureters in the bladder. The ureters are the tubes that lead down to the bladder from the kidneys, and the concern with the frequent urinary tract infections was that the infections could ascend from the bladder into the ureters and ultimately cause damage to the kidneys.

Darlene was a delightful baby who gurgled and smiled and never cried during the examination. I plotted her height and weight on standardized growth charts, and she was within normal range, showing that the infections had not caused any retardation of her growth. She was able to sit up without support and crawled without help. Her responses to stimuli were as expected for her age.

I began the physical examination and noted that she had a clitoris that was slightly larger than usual, and the labia were fused and looked like a scrotum. I palpated what looked like the scrotum and was unable to detect any masses within. I was looking to see if there was any possibility of testicles being found within, and I determined that there was not, but also considered the possibility that they were present but un-descended. In a male child, the testicles are originally located in the abdominal cavity but descend into the scrotum before birth. Occasionally this does not happen.

It is important to detect this early as the increased temperature in the abdominal cavity affects the testicles negatively and can make the person permanently sterile. Since this was before the day that ultrasound and DNA testing was available, I had to rely on my training in physical diagnosis by taking an extensive history and doing a complete physical. I asked the mother if she had taken any hormones during her pregnancy and if this sort of problem was known in any other family members. Her answer was a resounding "no" to all questions, and Darlene was her only child. I pointed out the fused labia and asked if she had noted this earlier, closer to Darlene's birth. She said she didn't think it was present at birth but was uncertain. This may explain why there was no question about Darlene's sex at birth and made it more likely that she was in fact a female with labia that had fused for a variety of reasons. In some cases, it is caused by the reluctance of parents to cleanse the area properly, occasionally due to their own inhibitions of invasiveness in that area. The resulting recurrent urinary tract infections may also have worsened the problem. The problem sometimes occurs a month or two after birth as the estrogens that the infant is exposed to in utero begin to wane after birth. Moreover, the fused labia could have been the cause of the recurrent urinary tract infections.

I decided to try having the mother rub some estrogen cream on the labia to see if they would open spontaneously. Surgical opening was a much less desirable solution because often that led to the labia fusing again. I saw Darlene about a month later and was pleased to note that the labia had opened about halfway. After another month of the estrogen cream, the labia had fully separated and Darlene had not had any more urinary tract infections. The parents were greatly relieved that surgery had been avoided and Darlene, her parents, and grandparents remained in my care for many years after.

However, this was not the end of Darlene's problems. Several months later, Darlene started to have recurrent cases of bronchitis in close succession. Although she always kept her cheery demeanor, the episodes were accompanied by severe coughing and high fever. Physical examination revealed that the infections were starting to cause her failure to thrive. I treated her with humidified air and antibiotics and in each event she recovered but became sick again just a short time later. I knew both parents were smokers as I could always smell it off their clothing, and although they were not yet my patients at the time, I mentioned at each visit that they should not smoke in the presence of the child. It is difficult for me to say to what degree they followed my instructions, but I suspected they did not in view of Darlene's recurring upper respiratory infections. After the fourth such occurrence in recent months, I now spoke strongly to both parents and informed them of the danger to the child's health of the child's recurrent illnesses, and I threatened to report them to the Division of Youth and Family Services if they continued to smoke in the presence of their infant as it was likely that this was making her sick. This warning must have taken hold, as I did not see Darlene for another respiratory infection for the next few years until she started kindergarten.

A few weeks later Darlene's mother, Deirdre, came into my office saying she wanted to quit smoking and asking could I help her. Since I was also a certified specialist in Addiction Medicine, I agreed to treat her. Weekly Smoker's Anonymous meetings were held in my office, and I suggested she commit to attend them. I also offered her medical treatment with ear acupuncture and told her that she would have to come to the office several times a week for that. Apparently she was familiar with acupuncture having had some treatments for back pain, and she eagerly agreed to this treatment. Deirdre attended the Smoker's Anonymous meetings regularly and came diligently for her acupuncture treatments. She was doing very well for about two months and was smoke free although she said her husband had not quit but at least did not smoke in the house any longer. At each visit she commented laughingly that she was gaining weight, and I tried to show her that always needing to stick something in her mouth instead of a cigarette was counter to her recovery. In addiction treatment it is not infrequently seen that patients switch addictions thinking that is recovery. Some people give up alcohol but then take pills to calm them, help them sleep, etc. That is not recovery as that behavior frequently leads them right back to their drug of choice. At each visit I would weigh Deirdre, and after two months being smoke free, she had in fact gained fifteen pounds. Now she wasn't laughing about it any longer, and she told me her husband was making nasty comments and constantly telling her he liked her better when she was smoking. At that point she had been weaned off her acupuncture treatments so I didn't see her as frequently in the office, but I learned she had stopped going to the Smoker's Anonymous meetings. Soon she stopped coming to the office altogether. However, several years later both Deirdre and her husband came back in for treatment again.

Addiction is a very compelling illness and often recovery is characterized by two steps forward and one step back. Eventually both Deirdre and her husband became successful non-smokers and continued to attend the Smoker's Anonymous meetings for several years and became dedicated sponsors to many others.

The Waiting Room

⊱◈⊰

All of the previous chapters dealt with experiences that I had in the examination rooms of my office. It might seem like a stretch of the imagination to think that there were interesting occurrences over the years which took place in the waiting room as well. But there were such instances, some happy, some sad, some terrifying, and some inspirational.

1. Josephine had been a patient of mine for about seven or eight years. She was now thirty years old, unmarried, and not a happy camper. She was markedly obese—five feet tall and weighed on the far side of two hundred pounds. She had never dated and lived with an older sister and her sister's husband in a small house near my office. I would see her for her yearly physicals and during the year for minor ailments. At each visit I would attempt to urge her to lose weight and

suggested several times that she attend meetings at a local Weight Watchers group. She would do it but not for long and with each relapse, gain even more weight.

She was equally unhappy in her living arrangements and told me that every night right after dinner she would retreat to her small room so as not to interfere with her sister's privacy. She worked during the day at a job which she said she hated as the other employees were skinny and fit young girls who she suspected made fun of her weight when they thought she didn't hear them. It was always distressing to listen to what she shared with me, and despite my constant encouragement to join groups and get out and meet people, I knew she was too inhibited by her appearance to do it.

One day I was detained in the emergency room and came to my office about forty-five minutes late. Although it was the practice of my office staff to call people if I was delayed, they were unable to reach Josephine and so she arrived early only to have to wait for my arrival. Another patient came there early as well as he was a new patient and the staff did not have his contact information as yet.

He had just moved to the area, having been transferred by his work to a new location into which they had just expanded. His name was Alphonse. Since the office staff was able to reach everyone else to tell them that I was delayed, Josephine and Alphonse were the only people in the waiting room. While waiting for me, they struck up a conversation.

After I arrived, Josephine was brought into the examination room. I immediately noted that her face was quite flushed and she was smiling from ear to ear. She told me about meeting that man in the waiting room and that he was so friendly and nice to her and that he asked her to go to a movie with him. I was pleased to hear this and share her excitement. I tried to keep our meeting to medical considerations but she was more interested in asking me about what she should wear and how to behave on their date. Our meeting was more like two girlfriends than it was doctor and patient, but I felt that at that moment Josephine needed a friend more than a doctor. So I attended to her medical issue and soon afterward she left.

When Alphonse came into the examination room, I apologized for making him wait. He told me he didn't mind waiting at all and in fact had met a lovely lady in the waiting room with whom he had a delightful conversation. His visit was just for the purpose of acquainting me with his medical history for which he brought his records. He was also quite obese and had a number of related medical problems. I told him I would look them over after hours as I was already considerably behind for the day.

Apparently Josephine and Alphonse (call me Al) continued to date, and several months later he proposed marriage. Josephine called the office to tell me of this and to invite me to the wedding. She said she would love me to be there with them since it had all started in my waiting room. However, when the invitation arrived I had to decline as the wedding was to take place in another state as that was where Alphonse's extended family resided. However, my delight was not lessened by hearing the wonderful news but not being able to attend the wedding. That was my happiest waiting room occurrence.

2. One evening a patient came in to see me for a cold. She was a lady who came in periodically with her three daughters. I always noted that she was impeccably groomed and learned that she was the executive secretary to the CEO of a large corporation located nearby. I would see her for her yearly physicals but only rarely, if ever, for anything else. However, this evening she looked quite disheveled and markedly distressed. When I questioned her as to what brought her into the office this evening, she said it was for a cold. I looked long and hard at her and then said, "Barbara, you are a very smart lady. You know very well that if I had a cure for the common cold, I would be in Sweden getting the Nobel Prize and not sitting here in Rockaway, New Jersey with you. Could it be that the cold is what is breaking the camel's back, and there is more going on with you?"

This question unleashed a torrent of tears, and Barbara then began to relate a story of suffering to me which had been going on for the past year. She told me she had been hospitalized with back pain and in the hospital had been treated with high doses of Valium, a muscle relaxant and a tranquillizer. Upon discharge after several weeks in the hospital, the valium was suddenly discontinued. She reported that she became extremely distressed with severe alternating anxiety and depression. As she was unable to cope, this resulted in a psychiatric hospitalization where she was treated with additional psychotropic drugs. That hospitalization lasted several months. After she was discharged she continued to be very anxious and depressed and so entered a rehabilitation facility where more drugs were continued. At this point she had recently been discharged from the rehab facility but was still being continued on drugs which she said were not helping.

This story took quite a while for her to relate while my nurse kept rapping on the door to tell me there was a room full of patients outside in the waiting room. I felt that Barbara was in desperate need of help and that I couldn't cut her short as we needed to come up with a plan as to how to proceed at this point. So I went out to the waiting room and explained to the people out there that I was busy with an emergency and was sorry that they had to wait. I suggested that if their problem was not urgent that they make another appointment, but that if they felt they needed to be seen, that they would have to wait but I would see them that evening no matter how late I would have to stay. Since many of our patients were blue collar workers and were docked pay if they took time off during the day, many elected to come in the evening. So, to satisfy the needs of the population, I had office hours three nights a week.

Not a single patient in the waiting room grumbled or reacted negatively to my explanation of what was making them wait. I assumed they realized that if they had an emergency situation, that I would be there for them too. I was moved by their understanding and confidence which pleased me to no end. I took it as a very positive sign of the relationship I had with them and knew I would always do my best never to destroy that. It was very precious to me. Barbara's story was a sad one but the reaction of the patients in the waiting room helped to buoy my spirits.

3. Since my office had space only for one waiting room, it was often occupied by a mixed bag of patients. We did caution mothers bringing in young infants not to wait in the waiting room but to immediately notify the staff of their arrival so they could be placed in our baby room while they waited. However, apparently one mother had forgotten and remained in the waiting room with all the other patients for her infant's six week well baby checkup. When I examined the infant, she was doing fine, growing well, and in good health. Immunization was not given as she was still too young.

However, several days later the mother called me to say the infant was running a fever and had a severe noisy cough and seemed at times to be gasping for breath. I asked the mother to place the infant near the phone, and when I heard her cough, I immediately suspected that she might have whooping cough. Since this is a medical emergency in an infant, I arranged to meet them right away at the hospital.

Upon meeting, my suspicion was confirmed, and I arranged for the infant and the mother to be taken by ambulance to a nearby hospital which had a pediatric intensive care unit where she was treated.

About five days later, I began to run a fever and had a severe cough which was accompanied by whooping. I was tested and it was confirmed that I too had whooping cough. As an infant I had received the full course of pertussis (whooping cough) vaccines but sometimes immunity can wear off or never be fully established in the first place. Different vaccines have different rates of success. I never knew why I was susceptible, but apparently I must have caught the disease from the infant. Fortunately whooping cough is not a medical emergency in an adult. I was sick for about two weeks but whooped for about eight more. After the two weeks of acute illness, I was able to return to my office but still had a lot of explaining to do every time I whooped in someone's presence, and needed to reassure them that I was no longer infectious.

4. I did relate in another chapter an experience we had in the waiting room when an irate father burst in yelling and

being very threatening. I had seen his son for the first time that day just a short while before, and after examining him, told the mother that it seemed as if the child was not growing properly and that studies to determine the cause should be done. The mother went home and told the father what I said, and apparently he didn't like hearing that. So, since he didn't like the message, he must have decided to kill the messenger. His behavior in the waiting room frightened all the other patients that were waiting there, including my office staff, and when I went out to see what the din was all about, he frightened me too. A staff member immediately called 911, and the police showed up and took him away. So, this was a terrifying experience for all who witnessed it, but fortunately the police came quickly and were very skilled in calming the man down and easing him out.

5. It was a policy of our office when people called asking to have their family join our practice to have them come in first to meet me and ask any questions they might have. So when a mother of six children called in, they were given an appointment later in the week to come in and meet with me after office hours were completed.

Since they were a large family of eight, I said we would meet in the waiting room as it was larger than any of the examining rooms and had more seating. Also there were books and toys available to engross the six children as I was anticipating a menagerie.

They all arrived at the appointed time, and we met and sat down to chat together in the waiting room. I couldn't help immediately noticing how well behaved the children were. Four of them took books to read and the two eldest held the two youngest on their laps and read quietly to them. I also noticed that the mother and father sat down next to each other and held hands. The mother was a pretty woman and was neatly and attractively groomed. I must admit that I expected a mother of six young children to look harried and harassed and unkempt. She wasn't at all. The father and the mother seemed very devoted to each other, and I felt as I observed the way they related to each other, it was a beautiful thing to witness. They brought to my mind a sign that hung on the wall of the newborn nursery lounge which is situated across the hall from the newborn nursery where family members awaited the raising of the curtains so they could see the new babies. The sign said, "The best thing a father can do for his child is to love its mother." I thought there was a wealth of wisdom there, and it was inspiring to see it in this couple.

I had seen too many situations in my practice, where, once a woman became a mother, she was no longer a wife. I was often shocked to see the changed appearance of new mothers with added weight and no effort to care about their appearance. They would come in wearing soiled sweats and sneakers, and even if the husbands accompanied them, all attention would be devoted to the infant and the husbands would be ignored except to do the carrying and settle the bill. Often, despite the warning of the dangers of doing so, the mothers allowed the infant to sleep with them, which could be dangerous for the infant but also did not make for a comfortable sexual relationship between the parents. I wondered if the mothers were using the practice for contraceptive purposes. In every case, the fathers were unhappy with the arrangement.

I saw too many of the fathers become accessories in these marriages, and too often this was a harbinger of marital problems to come.

The six children had previously been under the care of another pediatrician in the area. When I asked them why they were leaving his care, they told me that they were very much against having their children vaccinated and had never given them any medications. The pediatrician they were using told them that he didn't agree with them and that they should seek the services of another physician.

When they questioned me as to how I felt about this, I said that I saw my role as serving their needs and not their role to serve mine. I said I might not agree with them on everything they believed in and that I would tell them this when I felt that way, but I would only interfere if I concluded that what they were doing could cause a danger to life or limb. Since my philosophy about use of medication was that it should be a last resort and not a first one, I felt that we would probably be in agreement much of the time. I told them that I believed that humans had strong innate healing powers and that harnessing them should always be our first priority. They smiled and heartily approved when I told them this. I did point out however, that problems would come up when the children started school as certain immunizations were required. They said this was no problem as all the children were being schooled at home.

Several months passed before I got a call from the mother. She said that one of the boys was running a fever and complaining that his throat hurt him. I told her to bring him in that day, and when she did I could see this was a very ill child. Examination revealed a temperature of 104 degrees, large swollen lymph nodes in his neck, and a pus-ridden sore throat. I strongly suspected a severe case of strep throat and knew the boy needed immediate treatment. The mother had been treating him with tea and honey before she realized it was not helping and contacted me.

I told the mother the throat should be cultured but that I felt immediate treatment with antibiotics was necessary. She demurred asking if she could just continue with the tea and honey. I now had to explain the potential danger of strep infections which I was quite certain we were dealing with. I gently and patiently explained this to her while also pointing out both the contagious nature of the infection and the possibility of very serious long range consequences. I also emphasized the danger to the other children. I reassured her by stating that the treatment I was suggesting would have no permanent effect on the child. I also emphasized, however, that withholding treatment could be life-threatening. Finally she consented to treatment, and I gave him an injection of a large dose of penicillin which was to be followed up by ten days of pills given orally. Fortunately he recovered without event.

Although the parents continued to adhere to not allowing the children to be vaccinated, they seemed at least somewhat more amenable to medical treatment when, after gentle and patient explaining, they were convinced of its necessity. Since quite a few years passed before I saw them again, I concluded that necessity did not arise again.

I had many exciting, happy, and inspirational experiences throughout the years that I practiced Family Medicine. The memories warm my heart and brighten my days now that I am retired. It is interesting for me to note that, without having gone through my own very serious illness, which nearly took my life, I might not have had the many joyous experiences practicing Family Medicine that I had.

I guess every cloud does have a silver living.

Laurie

ೕൟ

I first met Laurie when she was just a few hours old. I had been called to the Newborn Nursery with the announcement of her birth. I knew the family well and had been their family doctor for the past ten years.

Laurie was the third daughter born to this family. The first two daughters were now five and three years respectively. Laurie's arrival was not planned. The parents were deeply religious people and had shunned the use of contraception and used the rhythm method instead. When the mother told me that she was pregnant once again I noted that she did not seem as happy this time as she had been with the first two pregnancies. When she told me this, I thought to myself of a joke we used to tell each other in medical school. It asked: "What do you call people who use the rhythm method of contraception?" The answer was "parents".

Laurie's mother had nursed the first two children but had elected not to nurse again this time. When I asked her why she had made this choice, she said it took too much time and she didn't have the strength. She also added that no one could help her with nursing, that only she could do it, whereas other family members could assist with bottle feeding.

Upon examination in the nursery, Laurie was noted to be a contented, placid infant. Without actually conducting a controlled experiment, I felt I could often predict the ultimate nature of a child by observations I made on them in the first hours of their birth. Some infants are easy to care for. They sleep a lot, don't cry too much, and are easy to handle. Others are very active, sleep less, often display infant colic, and in general are harder to handle. As I followed these children through many years, in quite a few cases doing their premarital physicals and blood work, I had many opportunities to see how they turned out. I felt my predictions were accurate in a lot of instances.

When Laurie was brought in for one of her infant checkups and immunizations, Laurie's mother told me that she was once again pregnant. Since she was already past thirty-five at this point, an ultrasound was done which confirmed that the infant was a boy. Since they already had three daughters, the parents were ecstatic about finally having a boy child. The father, who himself was a renowned athlete in the area, was especially happy and had already purchased a football and started to decorate the infant room with all his sports memorabilia and trophies. The birth was expected in about four months which would have made Laurie only ten months older than the expected baby.

Laurie had an uneventful childhood, and I only saw her for her regular checkups and immunizations. She was always cheerful and cooperative on all her visits, and, upon questioning, her mother never reported any problems at home or at school. When Laurie was brought into the office, she was accompanied only by her mother. However, when the youngest child, the boy, was brought in, he was accompanied by both the mother and the father and on several occasions by several aunts as well. It was obvious the son was getting a lot more attention than Laurie.

When my nurse told me one day that her mother was bringing her in for a medical problem that had her quite worried, I was surprised and wondered what could be wrong as she had always been so healthy.

When they arrived, her mother told me that the problem was that Laurie had not had a bowel movement for three weeks. Laurie was then nine years old. I glanced at Laurie when she told me this and noted that she seemed her usual cheerful self and in fact was smiling. If the story her mother related were actually so, I would have expected Laurie to at least look somewhat uncomfortable. When I questioned her mother as to her activity these past weeks, whether she was going to school and was physically active, and eating normally, her mother responded positively to all these questions.

I then proceeded to examine Laurie. If in fact she was eating normally but had not had a bowel movement in three weeks, I would have expected to feel "lumps" when I examined her abdomen, and her abdomen would be especially tender. Laurie was thin, so this would not have been a problem at all. However, her abdomen felt normal and upon listening to her bowel sounds with my stethoscope, they too were normal. If in fact she had not had a bowel movement in three weeks as her mother reported, her bowel sounds would have been quite noisy as the putrefaction of the stool staying in place and not being evacuated would have produced a lot of gas and would have created loud rumbling and tinkling sounds. And, of course, Laurie would have been in pain which she didn't seem to be at all. Since when I went to medical school and also in the early years of my practice CT scans and MRI's were not available, we were taught to make a lot of judgments on physical signs. Bowel sounds give a lot of information. They can be too loud and signal one thing, or absent and signal something else.

I questioned her mother as to how she knew about the problem, and she said that Laurie had told her this and also that she had taken to checking the toilet daily. I was certain something was seriously amiss with this story as Laurie's examination did not at all confirm it. I told her mother that my examination did not reveal any problems. This engendered a strong reaction on the mother's part, resulting in a reply which said that there was definitely a problem if a child did not have a bowel movement for three weeks. I could see that Laurie's mother had a strong need to believe this, so I did not immediately refute her belief.

I had learned in my years of medical practice that there are times when someone has a strong need to believe either that they are ill or that a loved one is ill. I didn't know what the reason for that strong need was in this case, why Laurie's mother had this need, or why Laurie had the strong need to have her mother believe this, but I knew from experience that the worst thing I could do was to just summarily attempt to remove that need. I knew saying "it's all in your head" would just send them from doctor to doctor until they found one who would agree with them that there was a serious problem here.

So I suggested that we hospitalize Laurie to do more studies and get at the root of the problem. This engendered a very positive response on both Laurie and her mother's part. They were both pleased that I seemed to be taking the problem seriously enough to hospitalize her and do further studies. Fortunately this was in the day before managed care controlled hospitalizations, and all that was needed was a doctor's admitting orders. More recently, before I had even finished writing a patient's admitting orders, someone from the Utilization Review committee would be breathing down my neck, questioning me about why I was admitting the patient and when I planned to discharge them.

Laurie was admitted to the hospital where I had ordered some innocuous studies to be performed. These did not include X-rays as I did not want her exposed to an unnecessary radiation. It was also before CT scans and MRI were available. However, I did order an abdominal ultrasound exam which had only recently come into use. It confirmed my suspicion that Laurie had absolutely no evidence of fecal impactions, or retained masses of stool. I also prescribed a placebo and told Laurie that I was confident this new "medicine" would help her problem. Placebos are not infrequently used in treatment, but when they are presented positively by a trusted person, they are often extremely effective. It has been reported that at least 75 percent of the time they do the job. That is why when experiments are done to test the efficacy of a drug, they are done as double blinds. This is so people don't know whether they are getting the drug or a placebo because it is believed their thinking will affect the outcome.

Laurie was told to inform the nurses of her toilet activities which after several days revealed no evidence of bowel movements.

We started to suspect that Laurie was flushing the toilet so no one could see her movements. So we decided to prevent the flushing without her realizing that was happening.

I called the maintenance department of the hospital to come up to her room and do something to the toilet to prevent it from flushing. The nurse came into her room to prepare Laurie for someone arriving to check the plumbing in the bathrooms on the floor.

The next day, Laurie was visibly distressed and came out to the nurses' station to report that her toilet would not flush. She asked what should she do but obviously didn't want the nurse to come in to inspect the problem. However, the nurse insisted, and when she did, she saw that Laurie had in fact had a bowel movement in the toilet. Everyone celebrated this fact and acted as if her problem was finally improving. No one suggested that she had been concealing anything. When I came on rounds to her room, I told her how delighted I was that the medicine was working. Laurie seemed relieved that no one seemed to be accusing her of making this whole thing up.

We kept her in the hospital a few more days, and since she was now getting positive feedback from both the staff and her family, she apparently no longer had the need to keep up the ruse and conceal her movements. The family was called in for a conference and without Laurie being present, was informed of everything that had happened.

The mother seemed more shocked than the father and kept asking why she would have done this. I put the question back to them by asking, "Well, what do you think she was getting out of all this?" The parents then looked at each other and both said at the same time, "Attention."

Laurie was the third daughter and the one born just before the long awaited and cherished son joined the family. She may have been the victim of a not uncommon disorder called "The Middle Child Syndrome". This is the belief that middle children get excluded or are even outright ignored in favor of the other children. These children are often overshadowed by their siblings, and that may have a strong effect on their personality development. As they learn early that good behavior doesn't give them the attention they need, they may often resort to delinquent or otherwise unusual behavior to get the attention they crave. The oldest child and the youngest frequently get the most parental attention and are often favored by the parents.

After acknowledging by both parents that the gain for Laurie in this situation was most likely her need for attention, they both resolved to attempt to work on this in their family situation.

Upon subsequent visits with the family, I learned the bowel problem had not reappeared and that Laurie was getting more attention not only from her parents but her siblings as well. When she was chosen recently to "star" in a school production, the entire family attended and then had an extended family party to celebrate her performance.

Laurie has become an exceptionally attractive teenager and was recently accepted onto the cheering squad of her local high school. The family attends all the athletic events which their son participates in, so they can at the same time witness Laurie's accomplishments as a cheerleader. I was told she became so good at it that she recently participated in a national cheerleading contest.

I was happy to see that the family was able to acknowledge the problem and act upon it appropriately.

Jake

❧◦❧

A major part of the work of the Family Doctor, who is the Primary Care physician, is the performance of the yearly physical exam. Barely a day goes by in the office when this does not occupy a large part of the daily schedule. The office staff always tries not to schedule these exams during our busiest time—i.e., flu season—and do them instead in the summer months. Nevertheless, requests still come in all year long. Patients need them for employment applications, for school and college entrances, for sports participation or renewed certification required by the department of transportation for driving positions. And then there are those who have suddenly recalled that they are overdue, or those who, experiencing a worrisome symptom, want one done ASAP.

161

As the physician for a large truck delivery company, I was doing physicals all the time for their drivers who were required to be recertified every other year and their managers who were entitled to have them every year. Since the company would quadruple their work force in the months before Christmas, and every driver hired was required to have a physical exam, we were especially busy during those months as well.

Having a physical exam was an important part of medical care because it presented an opportunity to detect conditions which, if the patient waited until they became aware of them, might be too late to treat. So there were many times when conditions such as elevated blood pressure, breathing problems, abnormalities of heart rhythms, suspicious skin lesions, or a prediabetic condition were detected before the patient knew about them.

Most patients came into the exam willingly enough, but often with certain restrictions which they exhibited. Some people were uncomfortable with nudity and didn't want to completely undress, and others were especially self-conscious about parts of their bodies. Many males were uncomfortable about undressing for a female doctor, and the reverse was true as well where many females were uncomfortable about undressing for a male doctor.

When I began my medical practice in a rural part of New Jersey, there were virtually no other female Family Doctors for many miles around. In time, as my presence became known, women started to come to me for their yearly examinations from quite distant areas. Some came from places as far as several hours away. Many had either never before been examined by a male doctor or had not been for many years. I began to realize there was a large population of women out there who would sooner die than allow themselves to be seen by a male doctor. These included women who had been abused, gay women, inhibited women, and markedly obese women. And so, to satisfy the needs of these women, I did a large amount of gynecological care in my office. I was often amazed by the long-neglected conditions which I encountered; women with large breast masses, women in pain with advanced cervical cancers, and women with masses on their genitalia. In one case, the mass had been present for twenty years. The poor woman was practically dragged in by her husband. Some of the conditions I could take care of, but many required surgical intervention and so I had to refer them. That was no easy task as they said they would not go to a male physician. It took some gentle handling and convincing persuasion to get them to continue their care. I often made advance calls to the surgeons' offices telling them what to expect and to make the effort to make the women feel as comfortable as possible. This was also in the day before a male physician was required to have a female staff member present while examining a female patient. I asked them to make certain another female was in the room to assist the patient.

Males often had the same reluctance about being seen by a female physician. Often I would do the care of a young male until he started to approach puberty and then his mother would tell me he would only go to a male doctor for his yearly physicals.

One day I got a call from a mother asking me to do a physical for her son Tommy who was now about sixteen years old. She said the exam was required for entrance to a school which he was planning to attend. I checked my records and noted that I had not seen him since he was ten years old, although I did continue to see the rest of the family including their three daughters.

When they came into the examination room, I noted that Tommy was very nervous especially when I asked him to undress. I tried to make him as comfortable as possible by giving him a large drape but with only limited success in making him comfortable. Nevertheless, I did not hold back on my examination which was to thoroughly inspect every part of the body. His exam was unremarkable although I did notice he had some central obesity and some mild gynecomastia or slight breast development which, in itself, is not terribly uncommon in teenage boys. However, I did make one very unusual observation. His testicles were not the size of a normal sixteen-year-old boy's. They were more like what I would expect in a boy of about five years old. I finished my exam and then sat down with Tommy and his mother and told them of my findings. I said I felt it was an unusual enough finding that further studies needed to be done to elucidate the cause of the unusual findings. The mother questioned me as to why this had never been detected before. I said that since I was not doing his physicals for the last six or seven years, I didn't know. They agreed to have it done, and I arranged for chromosomal studies to be done, which just required taking a swab of cells from the inside of his cheek.

The studies came back a week later, and it turned out that Tommy did in fact have a very unusual syndrome which would have led him to have quite abnormal development and would in fact make him become—technically—a eunuch. The studies showed that he had two X chromosomes and one Y. This would have resulted in a situation where he would have in effect been a castrated male. To prevent this inevitable outcome, he needed to get regular injections of testosterone to have normal development but would nevertheless be infertile for the rest of his life.

When Tommy learned he would require monthly injections, he became even more distressed than when he learned the news of his unusual syndrome. He had an inordinate fear of "shots" and I realized I would have to work with him to get over this fear as he desperately needed the hormone. So

I ordered vials of the testosterone and administered them monthly to Tommy and little by little got him to be comfortable enough to administer them to himself. Tommy did well, and his appearance in time began to change, and he started to look more like a normal teenage boy.

There were numerous other examples of males that had a reluctance to having parts of their bodies examined by a female, or even anyone for that matter. One patient who came regularly every year for his physical was Jake. Jake was a roly-poly guy with a terrific sense of humor. The office staff loved whenever he came and always looked forward to his arrival because he always brought snacks and made everyone laugh. He always made his appointments every year almost to the day so everyone knew when to expect his arrival.

Jake participated comfortably in every part of the physical exam with one prohibition. He told me at the outset that he would not let me do a rectal examination on him. I tried to explain why that part of the exam was important as I could detect early cancerous tissue and also check the prostate gland for any abnormalities before he became aware of anything. Nevertheless, he persisted and would not allow that part of the exam. This went on every year that he came for his physicals.

One day I was sitting in my office gobbling down a quick lunch while also going through a bunch of mail. I noticed a large packet and opened it expecting a display of sample office materials which frequently arrived. This time it was a bunch of sample disposable gloves. I noticed one glove was quite unusual. It had the usual five fingers but it had a long arm insert which reached all the way up to the shoulder. I was about to toss the gloves in the waste basket, but something prompted me to keep the glove that reached to the shoulder. I put it in a recess of my desk and then forgot about it for the next few years.

One year Jake came in as usual for his physical, and as always he brought snacks and created great hilarity with the office staff. However, when I started to get ready to do his physical, he told me about a friend of his that had recently been diagnosed with rectal cancer. And then he said "Okay Doc, you win, I'm gonna let you do that exam on me that you've been pushing me to do all these years."

At that moment, a light went on in my brain and I recalled that glove that I had secreted in my desk several years ago. I guess I didn't realize it at the time, but at that moment I realized that I had been holding it all along for this very moment when Jake would finally allow me to do his rectal exam. So I told Jake that I would get the supplies I needed to do the exam and left the room to retrieve the glove. Upon returning to the room, I placed Jake in proper position to do the exam and then, making certain he could see what I was doing, I started to put the glove on—all the way up to my shoulder. Jake was an African American man, and if it were possible for such a man to turn white, that was what would have happened. However, I was not so mean as to make him suffer with fright for long, so I quickly told him I had been saving this glove for him for this very moment, but of course had no intention of using it on him. It was actually a glove meant for veterinarians who needed to go in deeply in order to aid delivery of a large litter. Jake and I had a good laugh together and even hugged. Everything proceeded successfully after that. But every year after that Jake came in, he mentioned that glove and asked if I was planning to use it. It was always good for a laugh together and made for a friendly relationship.

I am proud to think the atmosphere in my office was always professional but still left room for humor, warmth, tenderness, and caring.

Iatrophobia

❧

Iatrophobia is a fear of doctors. The word derives from the Greek "iatros" which means doctor and phobia which means fear.

Iatrophobia is surprisingly common. Most people do not particularly enjoy going to the doctor. The reasons may vary for many, ranging from the long waits to concerns about bad news or painful procedures. So some amount of anxiety is to be expected but some people experience a level that is out of proportion and which progresses to outright panic. The panic at times is so great that it forces people to actually cancel, postpone, or avoid needed visits, vaccinations, or treatments, or to engage in endless worrying about minor symptoms which might require a doctor's visit. Many people that suffer from iatrophobia also suffer from a related fear, hypochondriasis, which is a constant obsession with minor ailments, lest those minor ailments require medical attention.

The anxiety related to a doctor's visit is for most people only transitory. Some amount of nervousness may be felt before the visit, on the way to the office, or while sitting in the waiting room and even in the examination room. However, it usually disappears soon after and is not so debilitating that it causes the person to avoid a needed visit. However, those that suffer from iatrophobia often experience a level of distress which is so great that they avoid the visit, or have extreme physical symptoms which make them feel as if they are totally out of control. These symptoms may make the administration of medical care either impossible or greatly altered.

Both the causes and manifestations of iatrophobia are many and varied. One manifestation of it is seen on almost a daily basis in the office. This is commonly known as "white coat hypertension". Everyone that comes into the office has their blood pressure checked by the nurse along with the rest of their vital signs such as pulse and body temperature. Blood pressure is often abnormally elevated by the stress caused by the medical environment especially when seeing the man or woman in the white coat, the doctor. Since this is a very common phenomenon we would expect the reading to be abnormal and therefore don't give it much credence. When it is noted to be at a level which causes concern, the patient is advised to acquire a blood pressure machine and take their own readings at home under more normal circumstances. Then they are told to bring back a number of these readings so that a determination can be made about what their blood pressure level really is under more normal and usual circumstances. I can say that, in my office, there was almost never any time that I would prescribe blood pressure medications without having the patient bring in numerous readings that they obtain on their own. I felt blood pressure readings should be taken during the circumstances that the patient is in most of the time rather than at the highly abnormal time when stressed out in the doctor's office. I have seen many times patient's discontinue blood pressure medications because they are not needed in more normal circumstances and they bring the pressure too low and the patient begins to feel terrible. Some have even reported that they passed out.

There have been a number of times when patients exhibited iatrophobia in my office but for different reasons and with different manifestations. I needed to be cognizant of their feelings and deal with them accordingly in order to effectively treat them.

One evening during office hours, I became aware of screaming that was going on in the waiting room. I excused myself from the patient I was with and went to the waiting room to see what was going on. What I saw there was a young boy named Charlie whom I knew to be about ten years old, who was struggling and being forcibly held by four burly strong men, two holding each arm and the other two holding each leg. When I questioned why they were restraining him this way they said it was because he needed medical attention and refused to come to the doctor. I had been caring for this young boy for a number of years and had never before seen him to exhibit such a level of anxiety about coming to me. We put them all in an examination room, and I came in soon after.

The men restraining Charlie told me that he had been sent home from school that day because he was noted to have "red eyes" which I could immediately see was a case of conjunctivitis. It is usually a very common and harmless condition, but because it is so contagious, the children are sent home and cannot return to school until they obtain treatment. I asked Charlie why he was so afraid as all he needed were some eye drops that wouldn't hurt at all, and he told me that one of the boys in school had told him that it had to be treated with needles inserted into his eyes. This frightened him so much that he determined never to have it treated even if it meant he couldn't go to school any more. I smiled and chuckled when he told me this, and I assured him it was not so. I had to make this promise to him about four or five times before he began to relax and the men could release their hold on him. The men said he was so out of control and so adamant about refusing treatment that his father had to call them to bring him to the office that evening. Charlie's father was a volunteer fireman in the town they lived in, and so rounding up their help at a moment's notice was no problem.

Charlie recovered uneventfully and every time he came to the office after that we laughed together about the events of that evening. Charlie became a stand-up comic at a local theater and so was a constant source of humor for me and our community. He told me the retelling of this story got incorporated into his "routine" and always was good for a laugh.

Mario came in for an appointment one afternoon at the urging of his wife. He said he would never be here except that he had agreed to submit to having his blood drawn for liver function studies because she was concerned about the amount of alcohol he was consuming. She was threatening to leave him if he did not agree to have this done.

I questioned him about how much alcohol he was consuming, and he said not much at all and that his wife was worrying for nothing and that he was only doing this to please her. I had long ago heard the joke about how to tell if an alcoholic is lying. The answer was "when his lips are moving." Alcoholics often deny or outright lie about how much they are consuming. And so I didn't put much credence in what Mario was confessing. Further questioning about problems at work or whether he had ever gotten a summons for driving under the influence were all denied.

He kept maintaining that his wife being a teetotaler was making a big fuss about nothing and that he was just here to please her.

I performed a physical examination on Mario and noted that he did in fact exhibit a number of signs of alcoholism. His blood pressure and pulse rate were elevated, and he exhibited tremors of his hands. His face was florid and marked by numerous tiny blood vessels. His body exhibited a condition called gynecomastia, or enlargement of the breasts, which is due to the elevated blood alcohol level causing increased conversion of male hormone to estrogen, a female hormone. Pubic hair distribution may be effected as well. I was surprised to note that his liver seemed to be normal in size and not especially tender.

Blood tests revealed a mild anemia and abnormal levels of pancreatic enzymes. However, his liver function tests were very close to normal. He was ecstatic to learn this, but I told him that he had quite a number of signs that the amount of alcohol he was drinking was causing quite a number of other problems. Excessive alcohol consumption may affect the body in a number of ways. It can cause the destruction of brain tissue which can lead the brain to shrink within the cranium and since nature abhors a vacuum, it gets replaced by fluid. This is the condition commonly known as a "wet brain".

Alcohol can affect the heart and cause it to function abnormally which may be contributing to Mario's elevated pulse rate and blood pressure. It can also affect the pancreas, causing pancreatitis which carries a significant mortality and morbidity. For some reason, in Mario's case, the alcohol was affecting all these other areas but not significantly affecting his liver, or at least, not yet. This was not the first time I had noted this in alcoholics. It is not known why some areas of the body are affected more than others.

I think I was able to impress upon Mario that his alcohol consumption was already causing serious problems, and he left resolved to discuss this all with his wife and obtain treatment.

So here I had a situation where a patient would have on his own avoided seeking treatment because he was afraid of what it would reveal, but only came under the threat of his wife leaving him.

Nils was an eight year old boy who had just emigrated to the United States with his family from Norway. His father was American and had been on a diplomatic assignment to Norway when he and Nils' mother met and married. They subsequently had two children: the boy, Nils, and a daughter, Margrit. They had settled in a home near my office, and the mother brought Nils in as he required a physical exam and immunization update before entering school.

Nils had had a bilingual education in Norway and spoke quite good English. I went out to the waiting room to welcome them in but immediately noted that Nils sat huddled on a chair, and his mother had difficulty in getting him to rise to go with her into the examination room. He rose very reluctantly, and she practically had to pull him in. It was not the first time I encountered children that were terrified of doctors.

In the examination room, instead of putting him right up on the examination table, I told his mother to seat him in a chair as I sat down in a chair next to him. We had a desk in the examination room as well as several chairs set there for when I was just conferring with patients and not examining them. I felt it made for a more collegial atmosphere for a discussion. I gave Nils a paper and pencil and asked him if he would write down his name for me as his name was unfamiliar. I felt this might help him handle his fear better by providing an activity for him and taking his mind off what he feared. Then I asked him why his mother had brought him to me and he said, "So I can go to school." I asked him if he liked school and wanted to go, and he brightened up and said enthusiastically, "Oh, yes, I love school."

I then explained that the school wanted him to come here so as to keep him and all the children well and healthy, and that sometimes that required having shots to keep them that way. He then said, "But I don't want a shot." And I asked him why not?

At this point the mother interrupted and said, "Oh, doctor, just ignore him and get on with it, and don't waste your time.

I can see how busy you are." I responded that I didn't consider it a waste of time and was enjoying getting to know Nils. I added that I felt it was time well spent.

Nils said he didn't want a shot because it hurt so much. I told him I understood that, but I assured him it would only hurt quickly and then stop hurting. I asked if I could show him on his arm how it would feel without using a needle. He reluctantly gave me his arm, and I gave it a quick pinch. He winced but then smiled. I then told him to do the same to me, and he reached over to pinch me. I too winced and then smiled and laughed. I then asked him if he would like to try my stethoscope and see what that was like. He nodded enthusiastically, and I placed the ends in his ears and put the other end against my heart. He grinned when he could hear my heartbeat. I then asked him if he would like to look in my ears to see what might be there, but also said if he wanted to he would have to sit up on the examining table because the tool to do that was on the wall. He agreed, and I gave him the tool and showed him how to place it in my ear. I could see he was beginning to relax and enjoy himself. I had some toy doctor's tools in a box in my office and promised him I would give him one after we did what the school required for him to attend.

I then began my examination as he became more and more comfortable. When I could, I enlisted his cooperation and that made him feel more mature and valuable. After that was accomplished, I felt he would then be reluctant to revert to being a baby about it all and wanted to show me how brave he was. At that point he allowed me to give him the "shot" which was not even accompanied by a whimper. He smiled broadly when I rewarded him with a toy stethoscope and a gold star.

I saw Nils and the family for many years afterward. His mother tells me how eager he now is to come to my office. I responded by reminding her that the time I devoted to getting acquainted and making him comfortable was time well spent.

Gerry had been a patient for quite a number of years but I had never met her husband, Marty. I just assumed this was another family where I saw all the members but not the husband. One day she mentioned to me that she was very concerned about him because at times he seems to "grab his heart" and have difficulty breathing. I asked if he has mentioned this to his doctor, and she said that he doesn't have a doctor, never goes to one, and that he has always been absolutely in terror of doctors.

I urged her to have him come in to see me and that I would be very patient and gentle with him and not do anything at all that made him uncomfortable. I said it would just be for the purpose of meeting and nothing would be done without his permission after first explaining everything to him. She said she would tell him this.

I heard nothing from him for several weeks, but finally the nurse told me the wife had called to make an appointment for her husband. On the day of arrival, I opened the door to the waiting room and called his name. He rose and crossed himself as he walked inside. He was white-faced and visibly sweating.

Once in the examining room we just sat facing each other on the two chairs I kept for that purpose in the examining room. We just chatted at first about non-medical things, and I then asked him why he came. He explained to me that at time he had difficulty breathing. I assured him that many things could cause that but I would only know after listening to his lungs. "Would that be okay?" I asked. He said yes, and I said I could do a better job if he sat up on the examination table. I also explained about the blood pressure cuff, how it worked, and how it would feel. I had the feeling that having his blood pressure checked was totally unfamiliar to him. I proceeded slowly with everything at a pace which I felt did not overwhelm him. I did not ask him to undress and listened to his lungs through his shirt.

I felt that was enough for that day, and so we returned to the seats and I told him that I didn't hear any problems with his lungs but probably some more studies should be done so I could say that with certainty. So with patience and non-threatening explanations, I saw the patient relax enough to agree to what I suggested.

He did return to the office and seemed more comfortable each time he came. And he did submit to all the studies I recommended.

Over the many years that I practiced, I saw many cases of patients that had neglected their health and suffered severe problems because of it. I saw women with sizeable breast tumors, people vomiting blood, and stroke victims that had never had their blood pressure checked. I was reminded of that every day I went to my office. Sitting on the steps most days was a married man with four children who, at the age of thirty-two, had suffered a severe stroke from which he had barely survived. He was left partially paralyzed with a severely limited ability to speak. I knew the family, his wife and four children, but I had never seen him as a patient. I only learned of what had happened when his wife came in one day to tell me and to bemoan the fact that he refused to ever go to a doctor because he was so afraid of them. And so, she was now the sole support of the family as he was no longer capable of working. They lived only a few doors down from my office and for some reason, when his wife was at work and the four children were at school he would limp out of the house and sit on the steps leading up to my office. I think seeing all the people going in and out provided some relief from his loneliness. Whenever I could, I would stop and chat some with him as well.

I have seen many patients with a fear of doctors, and I have no doubt there are many more that I have not seen. For some people the phobia is so great that it is crippling and they never get to a doctor's office. And so, those are ones I have never seen and know nothing about. And, if I ever do get to see them, often it is too late.

Salvatore and Marie

cๆๅๆ๑ว

Salvatore and Marie had been my patients for about ten years. I first met them when they were in their eighties. The physician that had cared for them had retired and since they lived just down the street from my office, they contacted me requesting to join my practice.

I first met them on a cold rainy winter day where the streets were icy and dangerous to walk. They came into the office well bundled up with bright eyes and cheeks. Because of the severe weather I suggested to them that they should have cancelled and remade their appointment on another day as they told me they no longer were driving a car and had walked over. They said, "Nonsense, we love the cold, and we support each other as we walk along the street."

The appointment they made that day was for both of them to be checked and for me to review their records. We had shortly before received their records from the physician that had retired. My nurse made these records available to me as they both entered the examination room, and I was surprised to note that there were only a few pages, whereas records I had received for elderly persons in the past were usually much longer.

When they both came into the examination room together, I asked if perhaps it might be better if I saw one while the other stayed in the waiting room. They both declined this offer saying they would not be seeing anything that they had not already seen in sixty-five years of their marriage. They told me they had married in Italy in their teens and had emigrated to the United States soon after. They had never had any children but had a large extended family nearby. However, at this point all the family members had passed on and they had only each other.

I had no trouble in reviewing the past medical records as both of them had never had any serious illness or hospitalizations. Subsequent physical exams revealed that both of them were extremely healthy, just not for people in their eighties but for people of any age. They took no medications and had normal blood pressures. What was especially surprising to me was that both of them had all their teeth and had never needed an extraction, a root canal, or an implant.

I complimented them on their good health and asked them what their secret was. They shrugged and said it was good eating, physical activity, and a strong faith. I also learned that Sal was an avid gardener, and although they had a very small house, they had a large garden and grew most of their vegetables. Sal also told me that Marie was a wonderful cook. When I asked her what her specialty was, they both replied together, "Lasagna." I said, "Oh, that is my favorite too." I probably should not have said that, because only a week later they delivered a large lasagna to my office which, after saying they should not have done that, I shared with the office staff.

I continued to see them for the next ten years during which time they never had any serious illnesses. They always came together and were obviously very devoted and loving toward each other. It was a beautiful thing to see how much in love they were. I marveled at how they helped each other and how they looked at each other as if they were still seeing the young and beautiful people they once were.

For me, it was a personally special delight every time they came into the office. There were times when I would see them walking together along the street, arm in arm, as they lived close to my office. Often I would pass Sal as he worked outside in his garden, and he would always give me a nice smile and a wave.

I have always found it to be an especially beautiful sight to see elderly people who were obviously still very much in love with each other. When I would see that, either as they walked along the street together or helping each other, performing tasks, or enjoying sharing things with each other in a restaurant, a theater, or a museum, I would always stop and watch and marvel at the beauty of the sight I was witnessing.

Sal and Marie exhibited this, and I always loved seeing them together. I must admit I didn't usually see husbands and wives together in the examination room, but with Sal and Marie, it seemed totally natural and it was obviously what they wanted. They were a team and were together in everything they did. They would not have wanted it any other way.

When I retired from my medical practice, I would often think of the patients with which I had long time associations. When I learned that Sal had died in his sleep and that Marie had died only a few days after, I found myself thinking a lot about their long-standing, enduring love.

When, in retirement I returned to painting, a hobby which had occupied my earlier life, I thought I would do a series which depicted my attraction to the kind of love that Sal and Marie had and which had always fascinated me. I might also add, at this point, that that also described the love that my husband and I had for each other. It was love at first sight when we first met, and that never diminished for the fifty-two years of our marriage.

So I embarked on a series of paintings which I have called "Ain't Love Grand" and have added it to this book which is, in large part, my own personal saga. I hope you enjoy them and are similarly moved by the love they exhibit. Because I believe that love trumps everything.